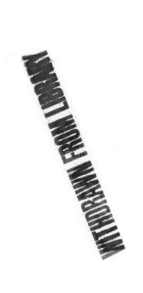

Simplified Diet Manual

SIXTH EDITION

Diet

Manual

Simplified

SIXTH EDITION

Diet
Manual

Iowa Dietetic Association

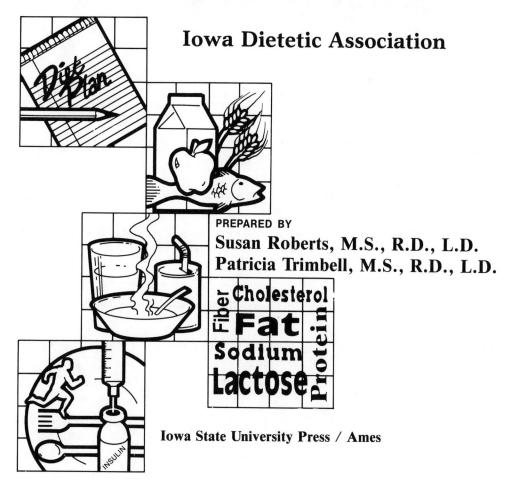

PREPARED BY

Susan Roberts, M.S., R.D., L.D.
Patricia Trimbell, M.S., R.D., L.D.

Iowa State University Press / Ames

Reviewers: Mabel Caviani, R.D., L.D.
             Mary K. Hogan, M.S., R.D., L.D.
             Angela Smith, R.D., L.D.
Content consultants: Kathy Buffington, R.D., L.D.
                             Emily Krengel, R.D., L.D.
Graphic designer: Jerold Best

©1958, 1961, 1969, 1975, 1984, 1990 Iowa State University Press, Ames, Iowa 50010
All rights reserved

Manufactured in the United States of America
⊚ This book is printed on acid-free paper.

First edition, 1958, *Second printing, 1958;* Second edition, 1961, *second printing, 1962, Revised third printing, 1965, Fourth printing, 1967;* Third edition, 1969, *Second printing, 1969, Third printing, 1970, Fourth printing, 1972, Fifth printing, 1973, Sixth printing, 1974;* Fourth edition, 1975, *Second printing, 1976, Revised third printing, 1977, Fourth printing, 1977, Fifth printing 1979, Sixth printing, 1980, Seventh printing 1983;* Fifth edition, 1984, *Second printing, 1985, Third printing, 1986*

Sixth edition, 1990, *Second printing, 1990*

The Iowa Dietetic Association acknowledges the use of the following registered trademarks: Bran Buds, All Bran, Finn, Kavli, Wasa, Triscuits, Rye Krisp, Cream of Wheat, Malt-o-Meal, Lactaid, Kool-Aid, Postum, Ovaltine.

The Diet Principles of the Liberal Geriatric Diet are reprinted with permission of Ross Laboratories, Columbus, OH 43216, from *Dietetic Currents,* vol. 8, no. 6, © 1981 Ross Laboratories.

Library of Congress Cataloging-in-Publication Data

Roberts, Susan, 1951–
       Simplified diet manual/Iowa Dietetic Association.—6th ed./prepared by Susan Roberts and Patricia Trimbell.
            p.   cm.
       Rev. ed. of: Simplified diet manual with meal patterns. 5th ed. 1984.
       Includes bibliographical references.
       ISBN 0-8138-1429-4 (alk. paper)
            1. Diet therapy. 2. Menus. I. Trimbell, Patricia. II. Iowa Dietetic Association. III. Simplified diet manual with meal patterns. IV. Title.
RM216.R63   1990
613.2–dc20
                                                       89–29225

Contents

About the Book

IN 1953 Nina Kagarice Bigsby, the dietary consultant to small hospitals and nursing homes for the Iowa State Department of Health, began a survey of diets that were being prescribed by physicians in Iowa. A trial manual was compiled and used for several months in ten Iowa hospitals:

Allen Memorial Hospital, Waterloo, Iowa
St. Luke's Hospital, Davenport, Iowa
Mahaska County Hospital, Oskaloosa, Iowa
Grundy County Hospital, Grundy Center, Iowa
Mary Frances Skiff Memorial Hospital, Newton, Iowa
Palo Alto Memorial Hospital, Emmetsburg, Iowa
Community Hospital, DeWitt, Iowa
Community Hospital, Belmond, Iowa
Story County Hospital, Nevada, Iowa
Loring Hospital, Sac City, Iowa

A special committee of the Iowa Dietetic Association was formed to evaluate the trial manual and to assist in preparing the manuscript for the publisher.

Hospitals in every state and many foreign countries now use the *Simplified Diet Manual.* Royalties from sales have gone to the Iowa Dietetic Association to be used for educational purposes.

The second edition, 1961, and a revised reprinting of the second edition, 1965, incorporated a number of significant changes based on experience in the use of the manual and on new information that had become available. The committee on revision included:

Dr. Marian Moore, Iowa State University, Ames
Dr. Margaret A. Ohlson, State University of Iowa, Iowa City
Anna Katherine Jernigan, Iowa State Department of Health, Des Moines
Mary Macomber, Iowa State Department of Health, Des Moines

A third edition in 1969 included changes and revisions that improved the usefulness of the manual and brought it up to date with current medical practice. Margaret B. Tait, nutrition consultant at the Iowa State Department of Health, did the major portion of the research and writing. She was assisted by a committee of Iowa Dietetic Association members.

The fourth edition, prepared by the Nutrition Section of the Iowa State Department of Health and the Iowa Dietetic Association in 1975, included changes in philosophy regarding peptic ulcer and gastrointestinal tract disturbances. Revisions in the Exchange Lists for Planning Diabetic Diets were added in a second printing in 1976. The dietary and nutrition consultants from the Iowa Department of Health who were involved in writing the fourth edition were:

Anna Katherine Jernigan, Director
Margaret B. Tait
Louise Dennler
Roberta McHenry

Members of the Iowa Dietetic Association who assisted in this revision were:

Dr. Wilma Brewer
Elaine Hovet
Ruth Huston
Mary Speer
Martha Spillman

The fifth edition was prepared by Patricia Kirkpatrick and Susan Roberts who were nutritionists in private practice, registered dietitians, and Iowa Dietetic Association members. The following Iowa Dietetic Association board members assisted with the revision and approved the fifth edition:

Mary K. Hogan, Chair
Margaret B. Tait
Patricia Moreland
Irma Johnson
Jane Baty

The sixth edition was prepared by Susan Roberts and Patricia Trimbell of Sue Roberts Nutrition Associates. It reflects needs expressed by Iowa Dietetic Association members and other users of this manual. These requirements led to revisions and reorganization to make this edition as comprehensive and useful as possible, consistent with current advances in therapeutic dietetics and guidelines for normal nutrition. Content consultants were Kathy Buffington and Emily Krengel, registered dietitians, and members of the Iowa Dietetic Association Publication Board, established in 1986. The following Iowa Dietetic Association members reviewed this edition:

Mabel Caviani
Mary K. Hogan
Angela Smith

The sixth edition was subsequently approved by the Publication Board, M. J. Smith, chair, and the Iowa Dietetic Association Board, Phyllis Stumbo, president.

The major changes in this edition are outlined in detail in the Preface.

Preface

THE SIXTH EDITION of the *Simplified Diet Manual* retains the basic purpose of earlier editions. In a simplified manner it provides a guide for the prescription and interpretation of diets or nutrition plans.

In the years since the first publication of the manual, many aspects of diet therapy have changed. One aspect remains unchanged, however: a patient's nutrition plan must meet her/his needs both physiologically and emotionally. While nutritional adequacy must be emphasized, the consideration of both these needs will make for greatest success.

Major changes in this edition include:

- Reorganization of diets
- Elimination of the following diets: Soft, Bland 1 and 2, Minimal Residue, Fat Restricted Diet (20 g fat), Cholesterol/Fat Restricted (200 mg cholesterol, 25% calories from fat), Severe Sodium Restricted, (500 mg sodium), Purine Restricted, 800 Calorie
- Revision of Sodium-controlled diets to be Low Salt [No Added Salt (3000–4000 mg sodium)] and Low Sodium (2000 mg sodium)
- Revision of Calorie-controlled/Diabetic diets to conform to the 1986 revision of the Exchange Lists for Meal Planning
- Addition of the following diets: Easily Chewed (Mechanical Soft), Dysphagia, Liberal Renal, Lactose Restricted, Gluten Restricted
- Renaming of the following diets: High Calorie, High Protein, High Vitamin Diet to High Calorie, High Protein, High Nutrient Diet; Liberal Bland Diet to Bland Diet; Postsurgical Soft Diet to Postsurgical Diet; Moderate Fat Restricted Diet to Low Fat Diet
- Major expansion of tube feeding/supplement list

The manual has been approved by five professional organizations: the Iowa Dietetic Association, the Iowa Department of Public Health, the Iowa Department of Inspections and Appeals, the Iowa Medical Society, and the Iowa Hospital Association.

We hope this latest edition incorporates the newest information in the field of nutrition and diet therapy in a way that will be useful to all those engaged in planning nutritious meals.

Simplified

SIXTH EDITION

Diet
Manual

1 Guidelines for Diet Planning

The Dietitian must provide nutritionally adequate diets as well as teach patients to choose such diets for themselves. An easy-to-use system that is flexible and dependable in providing the desired levels of the approximately fifty nutrients individuals need to stay healthy is useful in meeting this goal. A variety of guidelines to help with this task have been developed over the years.

The basic four food groups were developed by the U.S. Department of Agriculture in the 1950s. Using this system, foods are classified into four groups: milk, meat, fruit-vegetable, and grain. A fifth group classifying other foods was added in 1979. The Daily Food Guide: Basic Food Groups for Diet Planning, which follows this discussion, describes these five groups. The Daily Food Guide can serve as a foundation for planning diets.

The U.S. Department of Agriculture and the U.S. Department of Health and Human Services published *Nutrition and Your Health: Dietary Guidelines for Americans* in 1980 and 1985. These guidelines, based on research regarding eating habits and causes of diseases, recommend reducing the intake of fat, cholesterol, salt, sugar, and calories, and increasing the intake of starch and fiber. The *Dietary Guidelines for Americans* should be used along with, rather than as a substitute for, the Daily Food Guide.

The Daily Food Guide outlines the minimum amounts of various types of foods that are likely to provide adequate protein, minerals, and vitamins. This method of meal planning does not seek to recommend individual energy needs. Each person has internal mechanisms that regulate energy intake according to personal needs. The size of our fat stores, as reflected in body weight and appearance, make us aware when some conscious adjustment of intake and expenditure of energy becomes necessary. Therefore, the guide seeks to provide for nutrient needs, but does not specify energy (calorie) needs. Increased number and sizes of servings and/or addition of sugar and fats can supply needed energy (see Other Foods under Daily Food Guide). However, *Dietary Guidelines for Americans* addresses the maintenance of an optimum intake of calories while considering the consequences of high fat and sugar consumption.

Foods chosen for meals are influenced by personal preference and available resources as well as by nutritional content. Some nutrient needs are met primarily by one food group (calcium by the milk group, for example), while other nutrients (iron, for example) must be obtained through the combined contributions of foods from several groups. No single food or food group can provide the variety of nutrients in the amounts needed by the human body. Foods within each group are similar but not identical in food value. To achieve adequate nutrition, a variety of foods should be chosen from each of the original four groups.

The Daily Food Guide with the incorporation of the suggestions made in *Dietary Guidelines for Americans* will be the basis for planning the diets used in this manual.

DAILY FOOD GUIDE
BASIC FOOD GROUPS FOR DIET PLANNING

MILK GROUP

Milk is the leading source of calcium, which is needed for maintaining the bones and teeth as well as for many metabolic reactions. It also provides high quality protein, riboflavin, vitamin A, vitamin B_6, vitamin B_{12}, and vitamin D. Skim or lowfat milk and plain lowfat yogurt are the best choices in this group because they contain the important nutrients without added fat, salt, and sugar. All milk should be pasteurized and fortified with vitamin D. Lowfat milk should be fortified with vitamin A also.

Foods included:
Milk—skim, lowfat, 2%, whole, buttermilk, evaporated, dry
Cheese
Yogurt

Amounts recommended:
Choose number of servings as listed below:

Children under 9	2–3 servings (whole milk up to 2 years of age)
Ages 9–12	3 or more servings
Teens	4 or more servings
Adults	2 or more servings
Pregnant women	4 or more servings
Nursing mothers	4 or more servings

Count as 1 serving:

1 cup	Fluid milk or equivalent
1 cup	Yogurt
1 1/2 cups	Cottage cheese
1/3 cup	Dry milk powder
1 1/2 ounces	Cheese

Calcium equivalents:

Common portions of some dairy products and their milk equivalents in calcium are listed below. About the same amount of calcium is provided by each of the portions, but the calorie values are not alike.

1/3 cup dry skim milk	=	1 cup milk
1 cup plain yogurt	=	1 cup milk
1 ounce cheese, hard, semisoft, or processed	=	2/3 cup milk
1 cube-inch cheese, hard or processed	=	1/2 cup milk
1 ounce processed cheese food	=	1/2 cup milk
1/2 cup ice cream or ice milk	=	1/3 cup milk
1/2 cup cottage cheese	=	1/3 cup milk
1 tablespoon processed cheese spread or Parmesan cheese	=	1/4 cup milk

Fat content of cheeses:

Cheeses have varying amounts of fat. Those lower in fat should be chosen whenever possible. Processed cheese is higher in sodium than natural cheese.

Lower fat cheeses:	Higher fat cheeses:
Lowfat cottage	Blue
Regular cottage	Swiss
Ricotta, part skim	Cheddar
Mozzarella, part skim	American
Monterey Jack	Muenster
Farmer, part skim	Brick

MEAT GROUP

Foods in this group are valued for their protein, which is needed for growth and repair of all body tissues. These foods also provide iron, thiamin, riboflavin, vitamin A, vitamin B_6, and vitamin B_{12}.

Choosing a variety is important in the meat group because (a) only foods of animal origin contain vitamin B_{12}; (b) red meats and oysters are good sources of zinc; (c) liver and egg yolks are rich in vitamins A and D; (d) dried beans, dried peas, soybeans, and nuts are worthwhile sources of magnesium and are cholesterol free; (e) poultry is relatively low in calories and saturated fat when skinned; (f) fish is very low in calories and saturated fat and high in omega 3 fatty acids.

The amounts of the various foods listed are equivalent in protein content. Lean meats and dried legumes should be chosen most often.

Recommended intake from the meat group is 2 servings (total 4–6 ounces) daily.

Foods included:
>   Beef, veal, lamb, pork, fish and shellfish, poultry
>   Eggs (use in moderation)
>   Dried beans, peas, lentils
>   Peanut butter (high fat)
>   Nuts, sesame seeds, sunflower seeds (high fat)

Amounts recommended:
>   2–3 ounces of boneless cooked meat, fish, or poultry equals 1 serving
>   1 egg is equal to 1 ounce of meat, fish, or poultry, or 1/2 serving
>   1 cup dried beans, peas, or lentils, cooked, equals 1 serving
>   2 tablespoons peanut butter equal 1 ounce of meat, or 1/2 serving
>   1/4–1/2 cup nuts or seeds is equal to 1 ounce of meat, or 1/2 serving

VEGETABLE-FRUIT GROUP

Vegetables and fruits are important because of the vitamins, minerals, and fiber they contain. When the daily food guide method for planning diets is used, this group supplies nearly all the vitamin C and more than half the vitamin A. Other vitamins and minerals provided by this group include riboflavin, folacin, calcium, and magnesium.

Vegetables and fruits are low in fat and none contains cholesterol. The fiber in fruits and vegetables seems to be more effective when raw than when cooked.

Recommended intake from the vegetable-fruit group is 4 or more servings daily.

Foods included:
>
> All vegetables and fruits; vegetable and fruit juices (does not include fruit drinks or base)

Amounts recommended:
>
> Choose 4 or more servings daily including:
>> 1 serving of a good source of vitamin C or 2 servings of a fair source
>>
>> 1 serving, at least every other day, of a good source of vitamin A (carotene)
>
> Count as 1 serving:
>> 1/2 cup vegetable or fruit
>>
>> 1 fresh fruit, such as apple, orange, banana
>>
>> 1 medium potato
>>
>> 1/2 fresh grapefruit or cantaloupe
>>
>> 1/2 cup juice

Good Sources of Vitamin A
>
> Dark green leafy and deep yellow vegetables and a few fruits, namely:
> Apricots
> Broccoli
> Cantaloupe
> Carrots
> Greens—chard, collards, cress, kale, turnip greens
> Peaches
> Pumpkin
> Mango
> Spinach
> Winter squash (Hubbard, acorn, etc.)
> Yams, sweet potatoes

Sources of Vitamin C

GOOD SOURCES	FAIR SOURCES
Grapefruit or grapefruit juice	Honeydew melon
Orange or orange juice	Tangerine or tangerine juice
Cantaloupe	Watermelon
Strawberries	Cabbage
Broccoli	Greens—collards, kale,
Brussels sprouts	mustard, turnip
	Potatoes (with skins)
	Spinach
	Tomato or tomato juice
	Raspberries
	Yams, sweet potatoes

Note: Starchy vegetables (potatoes, corn, peas, lima beans, and winter squash) are listed in the vegetable group for diets other than the diabetic and calorie controlled diets.

GRAIN GROUP

Count in this group *only* those products that are whole grain or enriched. Foods in this group provide worthwhile amounts of protein, iron, several of the B vitamins, and magnesium. Whole-grain products are valuable sources of fiber and trace minerals, which refined products lack. The use of whole-grain products is encouraged.

Recommended intake from the grain group is 4 or more servings daily.

Foods included:
   Breads, whole grain or enriched
   Cereals, whole grain or enriched
   Grains, whole or enriched, such as brown rice, enriched or
     converted rice, barley, bulgur wheat, cornmeal, grits
   Flour, whole grain or enriched
   Pasta, whole grain or enriched, such as macaroni, spaghetti, noodles

Amounts recommended:

Choose 4 or more servings daily.

Count as 1 serving:

1 slice of bread

1 ounce (1/4–1 cup) ready-to-eat cereal

1/2 cup cooked cereal, cornmeal, grits, macaroni, noodles, rice, or spaghetti

1 tortilla

Tips for menu planning:

Foods from two or more groups are often combined in menu items. For example:

Meat and noodle casserole = Meat serving when 2 ounces meat are used

+

Bread serving when 1/2 cup noodles is used

On the other hand, the recommended 2-ounce serving from the meat group might be derived from two separate menu items. For example:

Bean soup containing 1/2 cup beans = 2-ounce serving from the meat group

+

1 deviled egg

OTHER FOODS

Foods other than those listed will usually be included to meet daily energy requirements (calories) and to add to the total nutrients and variety of meals. Sugar and fats are examples of foods that add energy value but few other nutrients. It is recommended that some vegetable oil be included among the fats used because of the polyunsaturated fat content and vitamin E contribution. Foods rich in sugar, fats and oils, and alcohol should be taken in limited amounts and adjusted according to energy needs. The use of minimally processed foods should be emphasized because of their important contribution of nutrients. If used, salt should be iodized.

DIETARY GUIDELINES FOR AMERICANS

Dietary Guidelines for Americans makes suggestions that can be applied when choosing from the four basic food groups and when choosing methods of preparation of those foods. The guidelines and some interpretation follow:

1. **Eat a variety of foods.** Choosing a variety of foods is critical to the effectiveness of the Daily Food Guide method as discussed above. No single food item supplies all the essential nutrients in the amounts needed. Variety in the diet is so important it deserves reemphasis. It maximizes the chances of including all the essential nutrients, minimizes chances of excessive intake of any nutrient, and minimizes chances of being exposed to excessive amounts of harmful substances, both known and unknown, in foods.

2. **Maintain ideal weight.** Obesity increases an individual's chances of developing chronic conditions, such hypertension, coronary heart disease, cancer, and diabetes mellitus. In addition, obesity makes even simple movement difficult, leading to inactivity. Both inactivity and excessive food intake result in weight gain. Menus should be planned to provide adequate nutrients without excessive calories.

3. **Avoid too much fat, saturated fat, and cholesterol.** Diets high in fat, saturated fat (solid at room temperature), and cholesterol increase blood cholesterol levels.
   Low intakes of fat and cholesterol are sensible. It is not suggested that certain foods be prohibited from the general diet, but that they be eaten in moderation or less often than is customary.
   Ways to reduce amount of fat and cholesterol in menu planning:
   - Choose lean meat, fish, poultry, dried beans, and dried peas as your protein sources.
   - Limit serving size if meat or poultry is protein choice.
   - Limit use of egg yolks and organ meats (such as liver).
   - Limit intake of butter, cream, hydrogenated margarines and shortenings, coconut oil, palm oil, and foods made from such products.
   - Trim excess fat from meats.
   - Broil, bake, or boil rather than fry.

4. **Eat foods with adequate starch and fiber.** When the fat content of the diet is reduced, the content of another energy yielding (calorie yielding) nutrient may need to be increased. The guidelines suggest increasing the intake of complex carbohydrates (foods containing carbohydrate in the forms of starches and fiber as well as other nutrients) to make up needed calories and to increase intake of fiber. Increasing fiber content in the diet promotes normal bowel function and may reduce the risk of certain diseases of the bowel.

   Ways to add complex carbohydrates to daily menus:
   - Substitute complex carbohydrates for fats and sugars in menus, such as using fresh fruit for dessert instead of pie or cake.
   - Select foods that are good sources of fiber and starch, such as whole-grain breads, whole-grain cereals, fruits and vegetables, dried beans, and dried peas.

5. **Avoid too much sugar.** Simple carbohydrates, such as sugars and products made with large amounts of sugar and syrups, provide calories but are very low or completely lacking in other nutrients. Since sugars promote tooth decay and since the body does not require dietary sources of sugars, minimizing their use is advisable. To avoid excessive sugars in menu planning:
   - Use less of all sugars, including white sugar, brown sugar, raw sugar, honey, and syrups.
   - Use fewer foods containing these sugars, such as candy, soft drinks, ice cream, cakes, and cookies.
   - Select fresh fruits, fruits canned without sugar, or fruits canned in light rather than heavy syrup.
   - Read food labels for information on sugar content. If the names sucrose, glucose, maltose, dextrose, lactose, fructose, or syrups appear first, then the product contains a large amount of sugar.
   - Use fresh fruits for desserts.

6. **Avoid too much sodium.** Excessive sodium in the diet is associated with increased risk of developing hypertension. Reducing the sodium content in the diet may also help to lower elevated blood pressure.

   Most food (except fruit) in the natural state provides some sodium. Additives, such as table salt (NaCl), preservatives, leavening agents, and certain flavoring substances, markedly increase sodium content. Many over-the-counter medications contain significant amounts of sodium, which should be taken into account.

   To avoid too much sodium in menu planning:
   - Cook with only small amounts or no added salt.

- Use spices and herbs for flavoring.
- Add little or no salt to food at the table.
- Limit use of salty foods, such as potato chips, pretzels, salted nuts, popcorn, condiments (soy sauce, steak sauce, garlic salt), processed cheese, pickled foods, and cured and processed meats.
- Limit use of frozen, instant, or prepackaged dinners, sauces, and gravies.
- Read food labels for information on sodium content.

7. **If you drink alcohol, do so in moderation.** Alcoholic beverages are high in calories and low in nutrients. The guidelines interpret moderation as one or two drinks daily.

2 Routine Diets

GENERAL DIET

Use: The General Diet is designed for persons who require no dietary modifications.

Adequacy: The suggested food plan includes food in amounts that will provide the quantities of nutrients (except iron for females) recommended by the National Research Council (NRC) for the average adult.

Diet Principles:
1. The diet should provide adequate nourishment, variety, color, and be pleasing in texture and flavor.
2. The quantity of food selected from each food group will vary depending on the energy needs and preferences of the individual.

FOOD FOR THE DAY	DESCRIPTION
MILK *2 or more cups*	Milk may be fresh, dried, or evaporated; skim, lowfat, or whole; used as a beverage and in cooking; yogurt
MEAT and MEAT SUBSTITUTES *2 servings* *(total 4-6 ounces)*	Meat, fish, poultry, eggs, cheese, dried beans or peas, or peanut butter
FRUITS *2 or more servings*	Fruits may be fresh, frozen or canned; served whole, diced, or as juice
VEGETABLES *2 or more servings* *(including potato)*	Vegetables may be fresh, frozen, or canned; served plain, in mixed dishes, or as juice Choices of fruits and vegetables should include a good source (or two fair sources) of vitamin C daily and a good source of vitamin A at least every other day.
BREADS, CEREALS, and GRAINS *4 or more servings*	Use whole-grain or enriched breads, cereals, grains; whole-grain or enriched pasta or rice

FOOD FOR THE DAY	DESCRIPTION
FATS *in moderate amounts*	Salad oils, fortified margarine, butter, cream, mayonnaise, salad dressings, bacon
FLUID *6-8 cups*	Water and other fluids, such as coffee, tea, fruit or vegetable juice, lemonade, broth, or soup
DESSERTS *1 or more servings*	All sweets and desserts

Suggested Menu Plan for General Diet
(Select from foods described)

Breakfast
Fruit or juice
Cereal with milk and/or egg
Whole-grain toast with margarine or butter
Hot beverage

Lunch or Supper
Soup or fruit or vegetable juice, if desired
Meat or meat substitute
Vegetable
Whole-grain bread with margarine or butter
Fruit or dessert
Milk

Dinner
Meat or meat substitute
Potato, pasta, or grain
Vegetable, cooked
Vegetable or fruit salad
Whole-grain bread with margarine or butter
Fruit or dessert
Milk

LIBERAL GERIATRIC DIET

Use: The Liberal Geriatric Diet is suggested for older persons as an alternative to more specific restricted diets, such as Diabetic, Sodium Restricted, Fat Restricted, or Cholesterol Restricted. This diet follows the basic guidelines suggested in Section 1. Older persons who do not require any dietary restrictions should be given the General Diet.

Adequacy: The suggested food plan includes foods in amounts that will provide the quantities of nutrients recommended by the NRC for the geriatric adult.

Diet Principles: (Adapted from Ellen Luros, R.D. 1981. A rational approach to geriatric nutrition. *Dietetic Currents* 8, no. 6 [Nov.-Dec.])
1. The healthy older person's needs for nutrients do not differ materially from those for any adult, with the exception of calorie needs, which are lower. For this reason, foods need to be chosen carefully to ensure adequate nutrition without excess consumption of calories.
2. The diet emphasizes the *Dietary Guidelines for Americans* with respect to sugar, sodium, fat, cholesterol, and fiber levels. (See Appendix)
3. If increased nutrients are recommended by the dietitian, additional sugar, fat, and/or supplements may be included.
4. Liberal fluid intake (6–8 cups/day) is recommended to promote gastrointestinal function and prevent dehydration.
5. Food may be better tolerated if served in small meals with regular between meal supplements chosen from suggested foods. No more than 14 hours should elapse between a substantial evening meal and breakfast.
6. Patients who have difficulty chewing or swallowing may need some foods, especially meats, chopped, ground, or strained. Meats should be moist and well seasoned. Be sure texture modifications are individualized and used only when absolutely needed. For further modification in consistency, refer to the Pureed Diet or, for easier digestibility, refer to the Bland Diet.

FOOD FOR THE DAY	DESCRIPTION
MILK *2 cups daily*	Milk may be fresh, dried, or evaporated; skim or lowfat milk is preferred; use as a beverage and in cooking; yogurt
MEAT and MEAT SUBSTITUTES *2 servings* *(total 4-6 ounces)*	Lean meat, fish, poultry, cheese, dried beans or peas, or peanut butter; eggs in moderation
FRUITS *2 or more servings*	Fruits may be fresh, frozen, or canned; prepared with minimal or no sugar (water packed; packed in natural juice or light syrup); served whole, diced, or as juice
VEGETABLES *2 or more servings* *(including potato)*	Vegetables may be fresh, frozen, or canned; prepared with minimal or no salt; served plain, in mixed dishes, or as juice
	Choices of fruits and vegetables should include a good source (or two fair sources) of vitamin C daily and a good source of vitamin A at least every other day
BREADS, CEREALS, and GRAINS *4 or more servings*	Use whole-grain or enriched breads, cereals, and grains; whole-grain or enriched pasta or rice
FATS *in moderate amounts*	Salad oils, fortified margarine, butter, cream, mayonnaise, and salad dressings
FLUID *6-8 cups*	Water and other fluids, such as coffee, tea, fruit or vegetable juice, broth, or soup. (Commercial broths and soups are extremely high in sodium.)
DESSERTS *1 or more servings*	Simple desserts such as plain cookie, sherbet, puddings

---

Suggested Menu Plan for Liberal Geriatric Diet

Breakfast

Fruit or juice
Whole-grain cereal with lowfat milk and/or egg
Whole-grain bread or toast with margarine or butter
Hot beverage

Lunch or Supper	**Dinner**
Soup or juice, if desired	Meat or meat substitute
Meat or meat substitute	Potato, pasta, or grain
Vegetable	Vegetable, cooked
Whole-grain bread with	Vegetable or fruit salad
margarine or butter	Whole-grain bread with
Fruit or sugar cookie	margarine or butter
Lowfat milk	Fruit or sherbet
	Lowfat milk

DIET FOR PREGNANCY AND LACTATION
(Based on General Diet)

Use: The Diet for Pregnancy and Lactation provides the increased amounts of protein, vitamins, and minerals needed by the pregnant or lactating woman.

Adequacy: The suggested food plan includes foods in amounts that will provide the quantities of nutrients (except iron and folacin) recommended by the NRC for the pregnant or lactating woman. Dietary supplements should provide only needed nutrients and should be taken only if prescribed by a physician.

Diet Principles: (For further reading see National Academy of Sciences, Food and Nutrition Board, Committee on Nutrition of Mother and Preschool Child 1981).
1. Weight gain during pregnancy should not be unduly restricted nor should weight reduction be attempted. The suggested weight gain for a normal pregnancy is 22–30 pounds. If excessive weight gain is a problem, the patient's portion sizes and intake of "extra" foods will need to be evaluated.

2. The possible harmful effects of caffeine intake on a developing fetus are not yet fully understood. Avoidance or limited intake of caffeine by the pregnant or lactating woman is advised.
3. Due to possible harmful effects on the developing fetus, it is advisable to avoid alcohol during pregnancy unless approved by a physician.
4. Women who are experiencing "morning sickness" or indigestion may find it helpful to eat "dry" meals, saving liquids for between meals; consume smaller, more frequent meals; and avoid spicy foods or foods high in fat content.

FOOD FOR THE DAY

PREGNANCY	LACTATION	DESCRIPTION
MILK *4 cups or equivalent*	MILK *4 cups or equivalent*	Milk may be fresh, dried, or evaporated; skim, lowfat, or whole; use as a beverage and in cooking; yogurt
MEAT and MEAT SUBSTITUTES *2-3 servings* *(total 6 ounces)*	MEAT and MEAT SUBSTITUTES *2-3 servings* *(total 6 ounces)*	Meat, fish, poultry, eggs, cheese, dried beans or peas, or peanut butter
FRUITS *2 or more servings*	FRUITS *2-3 servings*	Fruits may be fresh, frozen, or canned; served whole, diced, or as juice
VEGETABLES *2 or more servings* *(including potato)*	VEGETABLES *2-3 servings* *(including potato)*	Vegetables may be fresh, frozen, or canned; served plain, in mixed dishes or as juice
BREADS, CEREALS, and GRAINS *4 or more servings*	BREADS, CEREALS, and GRAINS *4 or more servings*	Use whole-grain or enriched breads, cereals, and grains; whole-grain or enriched pasta or rice
FATS *in moderate amounts*	FATS *in moderate amounts*	Salad oils, fortified margarine, butter, cream, mayonnaise, salad dressings, bacon
FLUIDS *6-8 cups or more*	FLUIDS *6-8 cups or more*	Water and other fluids, such as decaffeinated coffee, tea, fruit juice, vegetable juice, lemonade, broth, or soup

Suggested Menu Plan for Pregnancy or Lactation Diet

Use the suggested menu plan for the General Diet. Increase servings from the milk group by providing 1 milk serving or equivalent at each meal plus 1 snack. Increase servings from the other food groups also by either providing additional foods or by increasing serving sizes.

RECOMMENDATIONS FOR FEEDING NORMAL INFANTS

Use: These recommendations are designed for feeding infants, age birth to 1 year, who require no special dietary modifications.

Adequacy: These recommendations will provide the quantities of nutrients recommended by the NRC for the infant.

Diet Principles:
Breast Fed Infant—Birth to 6 Months:
1. Supplement daily breast feedings with vitamin D (400 IU daily), iron (7 mg daily), fluoride (.25 mg daily) to age 5 months.
2. Beginning at 5 to 6 months of age, solid foods may be offered.
3. A commercially prepared, single-grain infant cereal that is fortified with iron should be introduced first.
4. When iron-fortified cereal is being eaten, iron supplements are no longer necessary; however, vitamin D supplementation should be continued.
5. At age 6 months fluoride supplements may or may not need to be continued depending on the fluoride content of the local water supply.

Bottle Fed Infant—Birth to 6 Months:
1. Iron-fortified formula is recommended and requires no vitamin or mineral supplementation.
2. Beginning at 5 to 6 months of age, solid foods may be offered.
3. A commercially prepared, single-grain infant cereal that is fortified with iron should be introduced first.

After Age 6 Months:
1. After introduction of cereals, vegetables and fruits may be added. Introduce no more than one new food at a time and allow 2 to 3

days before adding another new food.
2. Small, frequent feedings are preferable for infants.
3. Canned fruits and vegetables, not specifically designed for infants, should be avoided due to the potential lead content of canned foods and higher sodium content of canned vegetables.
4. If preparing infant foods at home, start with fresh or frozen foods.
5. No salt or sugar should be used when preparing foods for infants.
6. Breast milk or iron-fortified formula is recommended for infants to age 1 year. However, when the infant is eating 200 g of solid food (6–7 ounces of strained food), homogenized, vitamin D fortified cow's milk may be fed. If cow's milk is used, a daily source of vitamin C is required.

DIET FOR CHILDREN

Use: The Diet for Children is designed for children age 1 to 6 years who require no special dietary modifications.

Adequacy: The servings suggested for various age groups include foods in amounts that will provide the nutrients (except for iron) recommended by the NRC for the average child.

Diet Principles:
1. The diet should provide adequate nourishment, variety, and color, and be pleasing in texture and flavor.
2. A sick child may regress in his or her level of performance, and this regression may progress throughout a long illness. For instance, a 6-year-old child may regress to the performance of a 4- or 5-year-old so far as eating is concerned.
3. Milk should not be drunk to the exclusion of other foods. If milk served with meals tends to reduce the intake of other foods, it should be served at the end of the meal or between meals. Whole milk is used until 2 years of age.
4. For younger children it is important that meat be tender, moist, and cut into strips or bite-sized pieces.
5. Young children like crisp finger foods; serve them regularly.
6. Excess fat can dull the appetite. Avoid fatty gravies, pastries, or repeated use of fried foods.
7. Highly seasoned foods are often not well accepted; use seasonings in

moderate amounts.
8. To meet energy needs of the individual child, larger servings of the suggested foods may be used, or additional foods may be added.
9. Vitamin and mineral supplements may be prescribed by a physician.

FOOD FOR THE DAY	DESCRIPTION
MILK *2-3 cups*	Milk may be fresh, dried, or evaporated; skim, lowfat, or whole; used as a beverage and in cooking; yogurt
MEAT and MEAT SUBSTITUTES *2-4 servings* *(total 1-2 ounces)*	Meat, fish, poultry, eggs, cheese, dried beans or peas, or peanut butter
FRUITS *2 or more servings*	Fruits may be fresh, frozen, or canned; served whole, diced, or as juice
VEGETABLES *2 or more servings* *(including potato)*	Vegetables may be fresh, frozen, or canned; served plain, in mixed dishes, or as juice Choices of fruits and vegetables should include a good source (or two fair sources) of vitamin C daily and a good source of vitamin A at least every other day.
BREADS, CEREALS, and GRAINS *4 or more servings*	Use whole-grain or enriched breads, cereals, grains; whole-grain or enriched pasta or rice
FATS *3 servings*	Salad oils, fortified margarine, butter, cream, mayonnaise, salad dressings, bacon
FLUID *6-8 cups*	Water and other fluids, such as fruit or vegetable juice, lemonade, broth, or soup

Size of Servings for Children

Food Group	1 Year	2 to 3 Years	4 to 6 Years
Milk	1/4-1/2 cup	1/2-3/4 cup	3/4 cup
Meat, fish, poultry, cottage cheese, or mild processed cheese	2 tbsp	3 tbsp	4 tbsp
Eggs	1/2	3/4	1
Potatoes or vegetables, cooked	2 tbsp	3-4 tbsp	4-5 tbsp
Fruits, fresh, canned, or frozen; dessert	1/8 cup	1/4 cup	1/2 cup
Citrus fruit and juice	1/4 cup	1/4 cup	1/4 cup
Bread	1/2 slice	3/4 slice	3/4-1 slice
Cereal/Grain	1/4 cup	1/3 cup	1/2 cup
Fats	1 tsp	1 tsp	1 tsp

Source: National Live Stock and Meat Board. 1987. *A food guide for the first five years.*

Suggested Menu Plan for Children
(Select from foods described)

Breakfast
Fruit or juice
Cereal with milk and/or egg
Whole-grain bread or toast with margarine or butter
Milk

Lunch or Supper
Soup or juice, as desired
Meat or meat substitute
Vegetable
Whole-grain bread with
  margarine or butter
Fruit
Milk

Dinner
Meat or meat substitute
Potato, pasta, or grain
Vegetable, cooked
Vegetable or fruit salad
Whole-grain bread with
  margarine or butter
Fruit
Milk

BLAND DIET

Use: The Bland Diet is used in the treatment of chronic duodenal ulcer disease, hiatal hernia, and reflux esophagitis.

Adequacy: The suggested food plan includes foods in amounts that will provide the quantities of nutrients (except iron for females) recommended by the NRC for the average adult.

Diet Principles:
1. The dietary plan must be as liberal as possible and individualized since patients differ as to specific food intolerances, living patterns, life-styles, work hours, and education.
2. A nutritionally adequate diet is essential if healing is to occur normally. The patient may need help in learning to choose an adequate diet. S/he should be encouraged to select the widest variety of foods s/he can tolerate since this increases the likelihood of nutritional adequacy.
3. Three to five feedings of moderate volume are most effective in reducing acidity and keeping the patient comfortable.
4. For reflux esophagitis a Low Fat Diet (45 g fat) should be followed in combination with the Bland Diet.

When a Bland Diet is requested, the General Diet is offered to the patient and the following procedures are followed:
1. Coffee, decaffeinated coffee, tea, decaffeinated tea, pepper, chili powder, broth, bouillon, caffeine-containing soft drinks, and alcohol are omitted.
2. Information is obtained from the patient regarding preferences and intolerances so that the diet can be individualized.
3. Three to five feedings of moderate volume are given.[*]
4. Acidic fruits, fruit juices, tomatoes, chocolate, and peppermint are omitted for patients with esophageal reflux or hiatal hernia.

---

[*]Normal weight: three feedings plus antacids; underweight or not able to take normal volumes of food: five feedings; no bedtime snack is given in order to decrease gastric acid production at night.

Suggested Menu Plan for Bland Diet
(Select from foods described)

Breakfast
Fruit or juice*
Cereal with milk and/or egg   **Midmorning**
Toast with margarine or butter   Milk
Beverage   Cookie or cracker

Lunch or Supper
Soup or juice,* as desired
Meat or meat substitute
Vegetable, cooked
Bread with margarine or butter   **Midafternoon**
Fruit*   Yogurt
Milk   Beverage

Dinner
Meat or meat substitute
Potato, pasta, or grain
Vegetable, cooked
Bread with margarine or butter
Fruit*
Milk

*If tolerated

HIGH CALORIE, HIGH PROTEIN, HIGH NUTRIENT DIET

Use: The High Calorie, High Protein, High Nutrient Diet is prescribed for nutritional rehabilitation of the patient following a debilitating disease or surgery. Food choices are made from the suggested foods of the General Diet.

Adequacy: The suggested food plan includes foods in amounts that will provide calories, protein, minerals, and vitamins in amounts greater than recommended by the NRC for the average adult.

Diet Principles: Lack of appetite is often a factor for a patient in need of this diet. To aid food consumption, consider:

1. Generally a patient cannot begin to eat a high calorie diet immediately. During the initial stages of this diet, portion sizes may need to be kept small. Increase size and number of servings gradually.
2. Some individuals eat better if food for the day is served as three small meals with three in-between meal snacks. For other patients a decrease in the number of feedings per day may result in a better appetite and increase total food consumption. Therefore patient's individual differences must be considered.
3. Although calorie needs are increased, addition of rich pastries, desserts, candy, and fried foods may decrease the patient's appetite for other nutritious foods, which are necessary for nutritional rehabilitation.
4. A simple addition to each meal may answer the need for increased calories, protein, and vitamins: for example, a slice of bread and butter or margarine, and extra glass of milk, or a bedtime snack of cereal with milk or cream and sugar.
5. If additional protein is needed within a limited volume or calorie level, an effective way of including additional milk in the diet is to add nonfat dry milk to fluid milk or to prepared dishes, such as meat loaf or mashed potatoes. The addition of 1 1/3 cups nonfat dry milk to 1 quart of milk will double the protein content.
6. Cream soups will add more calories and protein than broth soups. Adding nonfat dry milk to cream soups would further increase their nutritional value.
7. With heavy, high protein, high calorie meals, it may be better to serve a simple dessert such as fruit, pudding, ice cream, gelatin, or cookies.
8. Commercially prepared products may be used in-between meals or may be added to liquids for added nourishment and calories. Refer to Table of Products, Section 3.

Suggested Menu Plan for High Calorie, High Protein, High Nutrient Diet

(100 g protein, 3000 calories)

(Select from foods described in General Diet)

Breakfast

1/2 cup	Fruit or juice
1	Egg
1/2 cup	Whole-grain cereal
1 slice	Whole-grain toast with margarine or butter and jelly
1 cup	Milk
	Hot beverage

Midmorning

1/2 cup	Fruit or juice

Lunch or Supper

3 ounces	Meat or substitute
1/2 cup	Vegetable–raw or cooked
2 slices	Whole-grain bread with margarine or butter
1/2 cup	Fresh fruit
1 cup	Milk

Midafternoon

1/2 cup	Fruit or juice

Dinner

3 ounces	Meat, fish, or poultry
1 cup	Potato, pasta, or grain
1/2 cup	Cooked vegetable
1 cup	Salad–vegetable or fruit with salad dressing
1 slice	Whole-grain bread with margarine or butter and jelly
	Dessert
1 cup	Milk

Bedtime

1 cup	Milk
1 slice	Whole-grain bread with margarine or butter

HIGH FIBER DIET

Use: The High Fiber Diet is useful in the treatment of constipation, uncomplicated diverticulosis, irritable bowel syndrome, or whenever it may be desirable to increase volume of stool. Recent studies indicate additional positive benefits may be a lower insulin need when a high fiber, high complex carbohydrate diet is used in the treatment of persons with insulin dependent diabetes mellitus. Population studies indicate that a lower incidence of cancer of the colon and atherosclerosis is seen in countries where a high fiber diet is widely used.

Adequacy: The suggested food plan includes foods in amounts that will provide the quantities of nutrients (except iron for females) recommended by the NRC for the average adult.

Diet Principles:
1. The High Fiber Diet contains increased amounts of dietary fiber, defined as plant materials resistant to digestion. The best sources are grains, fruits, vegetables, and dried beans.
2. On a High Fiber Diet it is important to consume 6–8 cups of water per day due to the fluid absorbing properties of fiber.
3. For patients with diverticulosis, it may be necessary to omit foods with seeds or hard particles such as: popcorn, corn, peas, lima beans, tomato seeds, berries, figs.

FOOD FOR THE DAY	RECOMMENDED HIGH FIBER FOODS
MEAT and MEAT SUBSTITUTES	Cooked beans or peas, nuts, soybeans, and other legumes
FRUITS	Fruits, especially raw: apples, apricots, bananas, berries, melons, cherries, figs, grapefruit, oranges, peaches, pears, pineapple, plums, prunes, or rhubarb. Skins should be eaten whenever possible.
VEGETABLES (*including potato*)	Vegetables, especially raw: asparagus, broccoli, Brussels sprouts, carrots, cabbage, cauliflower, celery, corn, green beans, greens, lima beans, okra, onions, parsnips, peas, peppers, potatoes (white or sweet, including skin), radishes, rhubarb, sauerkraut, spinach, squash, tomatoes, yams

FOOD FOR THE DAY	RECOMMENDED HIGH FIBER FOODS
	Choices of vegetables and fruits should include a good source (or two fair sources) of vitamin C daily and a good source of vitamin A at least every other day.
BREADS, CEREALS, and GRAINS	Bran muffins; 100% whole-grain breads and crackers listing whole-grain flour as the first ingredient; bran-type and whole-grain cereals; unprocessed bran; use whole-grain flours in cooking whenever possible; brown rice; whole-grain noodles, macaroni, spaghetti, and other pasta
FATS	Nuts

Suggested Menu Plan for High Fiber Diet

The menu plan for the General Diet should be used, with the inclusion of the foods listed above (in each food group) that are high fiber foods.

MODIFIED TEXTURE DIETS

EASILY CHEWED DIET

(Mechanical Soft or Edentulous)

Use: The Easily Chewed Diet is used for patients who have difficulty chewing. This may be a temporary disability, which would allow progressing to the appropriate regular textured diet as able. Tender and easy to chew foods are served. Texture of the food may be altered by cooking, grinding, chopping, mincing, or mashing. The diet is prescribed in conjunction with other modifications as needed.

Adequacy: The suggested food plan includes foods in amounts that will provide nutrients (except iron for females) as recommended by the NRC for the average adult.

Diet Principles: This is textural modification of the General Diet or any appropriate modified diet and is designed to permit ease of chewing.

Suggested Menu Plan for Easily Chewed Diet

Select from foods for the day in the General Diet or any other diet. Follow the portion sizes for the appropriate diet using the textural modifications described above.

Breakfast
Fruit or juice
Cereal with milk and/or egg
Toast with margarine or butter
Hot beverage

Lunch or Supper
Soup or fruit or vegetable juice, if desired
Ground or very tender meat or meat substitute
Chopped, mashed, or very tender vegetable
Bread or crackers
Margarine or butter
Canned or soft fruit or soft dessert
Milk

Dinner
Ground meat or meat substitute
Potato, pasta, or grain
Chopped, mashed, or very tender vegetable
Margarine or butter, gravy
Canned or soft fruit or soft dessert
Milk

PUREED DIET

Use: The Pureed Diet may be prescribed for people without any teeth or for those who cannot chew or swallow more solid foods found in the Easily Chewed Diet.

Adequacy: The suggested food plan includes foods in amounts that will provide quantities of nutrients (except iron for females) recommended by the NRC for the average adult.

Diet Principles: The Pureed Diet is composed of foods that are especially easy to chew and swallow. Foods are chosen from the appropriate diet and blenderized or pureed to meet the consistency needs of the patient.

As the patient's ability to chew and swallow improves, the patient can progress to foods with more texture. Favorite foods of the patient are often best tolerated.

DYSPHAGIA DIET

Use: The Dysphagia Diet is designed for all persons with neurogenic or myogenic swallowing or chewing difficulties.

Adequacy: This diet is adequate in all nutrients recommended by the NRC for the average adult. Calorie level and food texture should be determined on an individual basis.

Diet Principles:
1. This diet requires extensive individualization and manipulation of food textures.
2. A high nutrient density diet may be indicated due to the high probability of inadequate oral intake in this type of patient.
3. Supplementation may be necessary until swallowing status improves.
4. Patients having neurogenic problems usually begin with smooth solids and thick liquids.
5. Patients with myogenic difficulties can usually tolerate thin liquids. Food textures will depend on level of chewing ability.

FOOD CATEGORIES FOR THE DYSPHAGIA DIET
(not food progressions)

THIN LIQUIDS*	Broth, coffee, tea, water, popsicle, gelatin, or any food having the same or nearly the same viscosity as water at room temperature
THICK LIQUIDS	Malts, shakes, nectars, sherbet, ice cream, cream soups, or any food having the same or nearly the same viscosity of nectar at room temperature
SMOOTH SOLIDS	Any pureed foods and foods having the consistency of pudding
SOFT SOLIDS	Canned fruits and vegetables, ground meats; bread is usually offered at this point

FOOD CATEGORIES FOR THE DYSPHAGIA DIET
(not food progressions)

SEMISOFT SOLIDS	Slightly more texture than soft solids. Begin addition of fresh cooked vegetables and fruits except those requiring a great deal of chewing. Meats are bite size.
REGULAR*	Includes all food textures including sticky, chewy, crisp, and combination foods

Tips for eating:

1. While eating, maintain an upright posture, at least 60 degrees. Remain upright for approximately one-half hour after eating.
2. Concentrate on eating. Avoid inappropriate conversation or distractions during meal time.
3. Place food on unaffected side of mouth.
4. Take small bites, 1/2 teaspoon or less, to reduce the risk of aspiration.
5. Eat slowly. The smell, taste, feel, and appearance of food helps to stimulate the swallowing reflex.
6. Try hot or cold foods. The swallowing reflex is triggered by hot or cold sensations.
7. Foods with combination textures are the most difficult to safely swallow and therefore should be initiated last.

---

*Not all patients will achieve a general diet or will be able to tolerate thin liquids.

3 Liquid Diets and Modifications

CLEAR LIQUID DIET

Use: The Clear Liquid Diet is prescribed for preoperative or postoperative patients; for patients with an acute inflammatory condition of the gastrointestinal tract; in acute stages of many illnesses, especially those with high elevation of temperature; or in conditions when it is necessary to minimize fecal material (residue free).

Adequacy: This diet is inadequate in all nutrients. It should not be used more than two days without supplementation.

Note: A commercially prepared "defined formula diet" may be useful if a clear liquid regimen is necessary for more than a few days or if the patient is seriously undernourished.

Diet Principles: This diet is composed of clear liquids. It is designed to provide fluids without stimulating extensive digestive processes, to relieve thirst, and to provide oral feedings that will promote a gradual return to a normal intake of food. Small servings may be offered every 2 or 3 hours and at mealtime. (Certain postoperative patients may be limited to tea and fat-free broth for one or more meals.)

FOOD FOR THE DAY	DESCRIPTION
FRUITS	Strained fruit juices: apple, cherry, cranapple, cranberry, crangrape, grape, orange
SOUP	Fat-free clear broth and bouillon
DESSERTS and SWEETS	Flavored and unflavored gelatin; popsicles; fruit ice made without milk; sugar, honey, syrup; hard candy
FLUID	Coffee, tea, carbonated beverages

32

Suggested Menu Plan for Clear Liquid Diet
(Select from foods described)

Breakfast	**Lunch or Supper**
Fruit juice and/or broth	Fruit juice
Gelatin	Broth
Tea or coffee	Gelatin
	Tea or coffee

Dinner	**Between-meal Nourishments**
Fruit juice	Fruit juice
Broth	Popsicle
Gelatin	Gelatin
Tea or coffee	Nutritional supplement

FULL LIQUID DIET

Use: The Full Liquid Diet is prescribed for the postoperative patient, following the Clear Liquid Diet; for the acutely ill patient; and for the patient who cannot chew or swallow solid or pureed food. It may be prescribed to supplement a tube feeding.

Adequacy: Depending upon the amount and choice of food eaten, this diet will tend to be low in protein, calories, iron, thiamin, and niacin. It is recommended for temporary use only. Vitamin and mineral supplements should be ordered if a patient remains on the diet for more than 2 days.

Diet Principles: The Full Liquid Diet includes foods that are liquid at body temperature and tolerated by the patient.

FOOD FOR THE DAY	DESCRIPTION
MILK *4-6 cups*	As a beverage and in cooking; milk in milk drinks, such as eggnog, milkshake, or malted milk; in strained cream soups; yogurt without fruit *Note:* Do not serve raw egg. Use blended baked custard, soft custard with added milk, or a commercial mixture that is pasteurized.
MEAT and MEAT SUBSTITUTES *4-6 ounces*	Eggs in eggnog, soft custard; pureed meat added to broth or cream soup
VEGETABLES *(including potato)* *2 or more servings*	Potato, strained in cream soups; other mild-flavored vegetables, such as asparagus, carrots, green beans, peas, spinach, strained and combined with clear broth, cream soup, plain or flavored gelatin; vegetable juices
FRUITS *2 or more servings*	Citrus and other fruit juices; pureed fruit without seeds
BREADS, CEREALS, and GRAINS *1 or more servings*	Refined or strained cooked cereals that have been thinned with hot milk or hot half and half
FATS *4 servings*	Fortified margarine, butter, and cream
FLUID	Coffee, tea, carbonated beverages
OTHER	Broth or strained cream soup combined with allowed strained vegetables Soft or baked custard; flavored and unflavored gelatin; plain ice cream; pudding; sherbet; popsicles Flavorings and mild spices in moderation Nutritional supplements

Suggested Menu Plan for Full Liquid Diet
(Select from foods described)

Breakfast
Fruit juice
Cereal gruel; with cream, sugar
Milk or milk beverage

Lunch or Supper
Soup*
Pureed fruit
Fruit juice
Dessert
Milk or milk beverage

Dinner
Soup*
Pureed fruit
Yogurt
Milk or milk beverage

Between-meal Nourishments
Milk or milk beverage
Fruit juice
Pureed fruit
Yogurt

*Soups may be fortified with dry milk, pureed meat and vegetables, and a fat serving.

POSTSURGICAL DIET

Use: The Postsurgical Diet is prescribed when it is decided the postsurgical patient is ready to have some whole foods but is not yet ready for a routine diet.

Adequacy: Depending upon the amount and choice of food eaten, this diet will tend to be low in protein, calories, iron, thiamin, and niacin. It is recommended for temporary use only.

Diet Principles: In addition to foods allowed on the Full Liquid Diet the patient may have poached, soft cooked, or scrambled eggs; cottage cheese; baked (no skin), boiled, mashed, or creamed potatoes; refined, cooked cereals; quick-type oatmeal; toasted white bread; soda crackers. Other foods from a routine diet may be added as the patient is able to tolerate them.

TUBE FEEDING

Use: A tube feeding may be prescribed for patients who are physically or psychologically unable to take food by mouth in amounts that will support adequate nutrition. Some of the described feedings may also be used as oral supplements to supply additional calories and/or other nutrients to patients who are able to consume some food by mouth. Tube feedings should be administered under the close supervision of a physician and monitored by a registered dietitian.

Adequacy: Some tube feedings will be nutritionally adequate when given in recommended amounts, but it is important to evaluate each patient individually.

Diet Principles:
1. Selection–Choice of enteral feeding product depends upon the medical and nutritional needs of the patient as determined by the physician and the dietitian. In addition to lactose-free standard formulas, there are those specifically designed for digestive and absorptive disorders, stress, trauma, and renal or hepatic disease. Availability of a specific formula will vary among institutions.
2. Administration–Access to the stomach or small intestine is gained via a very small diameter, flexible feeding tube. The tube may be placed naso-gastrically, naso-jejunally, or via esophagostomy, gastrostomy, or jejunostomy. Formula is delivered through the tube by gravity flow or by use of a metered pump. The concentration, rate, and volume of formula given depends upon individual factors, such as nutritional

status, body size, and type of formula. The feeding is initiated at a slow rate and/or a reduced concentration usually half strength or 300 mOsm/kg water. It is gradually advanced as tolerated to the predetermined rate and strength necessary to meet nutritional needs. Free water is provided at the rate of 25% of total volume of full strength formula. A multivitamin-mineral supplement is needed if volume of formula does not meet the patient's RDAs.

3. Complications—The major complications of tube feeding include diarrhea, constipation, aspiration, electrolyte imbalance, dehydration, glycosuria, and azotemia. Frequent monitoring of hydration status, residual volume in stomach, blood and urine chemistries, and physical signs is important in avoiding complications. Meticulous care in selecting, mixing, handling, storing, and administering feedings is essential.

TABLE OF PRODUCTS: COMMERCIAL SUPPLEMENTAL OR TUBE FEEDINGS

Formula	Form/Mixing medium	Volume (ml) necessary to meet adult RDA	Calories/ml	For Each 1000 ml				
				Protein (g)	Carbohydrate (g)	Fat (g)	NA (mg)	K (mg)
MILK BASED:								
Forta Shake (Ross)	Powder Mix w/whole milk	960	1.20	71	154	33	1000	3375
Instant Breakfast (Carnation)	Powder Mix w/whole milk	1200	1.04	56	126	33	1008	2954
Meritene (Sandoz)	Liquid Ready to serve	1250	1.0	58	110	32	880	1600
Meritene (Sandoz)	Powder Mix w/whole milk	1040	1.0	69	119	34	1100	2800
Sustacal (Mead-Johnson)	Powder Mix w/whole milk	800	1.33	77	180	34	1200	3400
Sustacal Pudding (Mead-Johnson)	Pudding Ready to serve	—	240[a]	7[a]	32[a]	10[a]	120[a]	320[a]
Sustagen (Mead-Johnson)	Powder Mix w/water	1030	1.7	112	312	16	1270	3380
MEAT BASED:								
Compleat-Regular (Sandoz)	Liquid Ready to serve	1500	1.07	43	128	43	1300	1400
Vitaneed (Chesebrough-Pond's)	Liquid Ready to serve	2000	1.0	35	125	40	500	1250
LACTOSE-FREE:								
Compleat-Modified (Sandoz)	Liquid Ready to serve	1500	1.07	43	141	37	670	1400
Enrich (Ross)	Liquid Ready to serve	1391	1.10	40	162	37	845	1564

Note: — = does not meet RDA

TABLE OF PRODUCTS: COMMERCIAL SUPPLEMENTAL OR TUBE FEEDINGS (continued)

| Formula | Form/Mixing medium | Volume (ml) necessary to meet adult RDA | Calories/ml | For Each 1000 ml | | | | |
				Protein (g)	Carbohydrate (g)	Fat (g)	NA (mg)	K (mg)
Ensure (Ross)	Liquid Ready to serve	1887	1.06	37	145	37	845	1564
Ensure HN (Ross)	Liquid Ready to serve	1320	1.06	44	141	36	930	1564
Ensure-Plus (Ross)	Liquid Ready to serve	1600	1.5	55	200	53	1141	2113
Ensure-Plus HN (Ross)	Liquid Ready to serve	947	1.5	63	200	50	1184	1818
Forta Pudding (Ross)	Powder Mix w/water	—	250[b]	9[b]	34[b]	9[b]	210[b]	350[b]
Fortison (Chesebrough-Pond's)	Liquid Ready to serve	2000	1.0	35	125	40	500	1250
Isocal (Mead-Johnson)	Liquid Ready to serve	1892	1.06	34	133	44	530	1320
Isocal HCN (Mead-Johnson)	Liquid Ready to serve	1500	2.0	75	225	91	800	1400
Isotein HN (Sandoz)	Powder Mix w/water	1770	1.2	68	156	34	620	1070
Magnacal (Chesebrough-Pond's)	Liquid Ready to serve	1000	2.0	70	250	80	1000	1250
Osmolite (Ross)	Liquid Ready to serve	1887	1.06	37	145	39	634	1014
Osmolite HN (Ross)	Liquid Ready to serve	1320	1.06	44	141	37	930	1564
Precision Isotonic (Sandoz)	Powder Mix w/water	1560	1.0	29	144	30	770	960
Pulmocare (Ross)	Liquid Ready to serve	960	1.5	63	106	92	1310	1902

TABLE OF PRODUCTS: COMMERCIAL SUPPLEMENTAL OR TUBE FEEDINGS (continued)

Formula	Form/Mixing medium	Volume (ml) necessary to meet adult RDA	Calories/ml	For Each 1000 ml				
				Protein (g)	Carbohydrate (g)	Fat (g)	NA (mg)	K (mg)
Resource (Sandoz)	Instant cystals Mix w/water	1896	1.06	37	145	37	850	1560
Sustacal (Mead-Johnson)	Liquid Ready to serve	1080	1.0	61	140	23	940	2080
Sustacal HC (Mead-Johnson)	Liquid Ready to serve	1200	1.5	61	190	58	840	1480
Traumacal (Mead-Johnson)	Liquid Ready to serve	2000	1.5	82.5	142.5	68.5	1200	1400
Travasorb (Travenol)	Liquid Ready to serve	1896	1.06	35	136	35	738	1266
Travasorb HN (Travenol)	Powder Mix w/water	2000	1.0	45	175	13	920	1170
Travasorb MCT (Travenol)	Powder Mix w/water	2000	1.0	49	123	33	350	1740
Travasorb Standard (Travenol)	Powder Mix w/water	2000	1.0	30	190	13	920	1170
TwoCal HN (Ross)	Liquid Ready to serve	950	2.0	83	216	90.5	1052	2316
DEFINED FORMULA PRODUCTS-VERY LOW RESIDUE:								
Citrotein (Sandoz)	Powder Mix w/water	1270	0.7	41	122	2	710	710
Ross SLD (Ross)	Powder Mix w/water	1200	0.8	37.5	137	0.5	833	833
Precision HND (Sandoz)	Powder Mix w/water	2850	1.1	44	216	1	980	910

TABLE OF PRODUCTS: COMMERCIAL SUPPLEMENTAL OR TUBE FEEDINGS (continued)

Formula	Form/Mixing medium	Volume (ml) necessary to meet adult RDA	Calories/ml	For Each 1000 ml				
				Protein (g)	Carbohydrate (g)	Fat (g)	NA (mg)	K (mg)
Precision LR (Sandoz)	Powder Mix w/water	1710	1.1	26	248	2	700	880
Vital HN (Ross)	Powder Mix w/water	1500	1.0	42	185	11	467	1333
DEFINED FORMULA ELEMENTAL:								
Amin-Aid (Kendall McGaw)	Powder Mix w/water	—	2.0	19	366	46	<345	<235
Criticare HN (Mead-Johnson)	Liquid Ready to serve	1892	1.06	38	222	3	630	1320
Hepatic-Aid II (Kendall McGaw)	Powder Mix w/water	—	1.1	44	169	36	<345	<235
Stresstein (Sandoz)	Powder Mix w/water	2000	1.2	70	170	28	650	1100
Travasorb Hepatic (Travenol)	Powder Mix w/water	2100	1.1	29	209	14	445	1140
Travasorb Renal (Travenol)	Powder Mix w/water	2100	1.35	23	271	18	0	0
Trasvasorb Standard (Travenol)	Powder Mix w/water	2000	1.0	30	190	13	920	1170
Vivonex HN (Norwich-Eaton)	Powder Mix w/water	3000	1.0	46	210	1	529	1173
Vivonex Standard (Norwich-Eaton)	Powder Mix w/water	1800	1.0	20	231	1.5	468	1172
Vivonex TEN (Norwich-Eaton)	Powder Mix w/water	2000	1.0	38	206	3	460	782

TABLE OF PRODUCTS: COMMERCIAL SUPPLEMENTAL OR TUBE FEEDINGS (continued)

Formula	Form	Calories per ml or gram	For Each 1000 Calories				
			Protein (g)	Carbohydrate (g)	Fat (g)	NA (mg)	K (mg)
PROTEIN SUPPLEMENTS:							
Casec (Mead-Johnson)	Powder	3.7	238	0	5	410	27
Nutrisource Protein (Sandoz)	Powder	4.0	188	17	21	670	1414
ProMod (Ross)	Powder	4.2	179	24	21	460	2300
Propac (Chesebrough-Pond's)	Powder	4.0	192	13	20	580	1300
Nonfat Dry Milk	Powder Instant	3.6	98	146	2	1531	4761
CARBOHYDRATE SUPPLEMENTS:							
Moducal (Mead-Johnson)	Powder	3.8	0	250	0	180	10
Nutrisource Carbohydrate (Sandoz)	Liquid	3.2	0	250	0	6	4
Polycose Liquid (Ross)	Liquid	2.0	0	250	0	290	100
Sumacal (Chesebrough-Pond's)	Powder	3.8	0	250	0	260	N/A
Corn Syrup	Liquid	3.8	0	260	0	526	18
FAT SUPPLEMENTS:							
MCT oil (Mead-Johnson)	Liquid	7.7	0	0	122	0	0
Microlipid (Chesebrough-Pond's)	Liquid	4.5	0	0	111	0	0

TABLE OF PRODUCTS: COMMERCIAL SUPPLEMENTAL OR TUBE FEEDINGS (continued)

Formula	Form	Calories per ml or gram	For Each 1000 Calories				
			Protein (g)	Carbohydrate (g)	Fat (g)	NA (mg)	K (mg)
Nutrisource Lipid-Long Chain Triglycerides (Sandoz)	Liquid	2.2	0	0	111	0	0
Nutrisource Lipid-Medium Chain Triglycerides (Sandoz)	Liquid	2.0	0	0	120	0	0
Vegetable oil	Liquid	8.0	0	0	113	0	0

Note: — = does not meet RDA
[a] Per 5 oz serving
[b] Per single serving

43

4 Diabetic/ Calorie-controlled Diets

DIABETIC DIET

Use: The Diabetic Diet is an outline for planning a diet with a diabetic patient.

Adequacy: The suggested food plan includes foods in amounts that will provide the quantities of nutrients (except iron for females) recommended by the NRC for the average adult.

Diet Principles:
1. *Individualization.* Individualization of treatment for patients with specific metabolic abnormalities associated with the diabetic state is essential and must be emphasized. To be practical and effective, the dietary program and teaching plan must be based upon evaluation of the needs, abilities, and resources of the individual patient. Reinforcement of teaching and encouragement are usually necessary over an extended period of time.
2. *Total Calories.* An important objective in dietary treatment of diabetic patients is attaining ideal body weight. For the obese patient, calorie intake must be less than expenditure so that the individual can achieve weight loss to the ideal level. For the diabetic person of ideal weight, calorie intake must match expenditure to maintain ideal weight. For the person below ideal weight, calorie intake must allow for appropriate weight gain, and, in the case of the young, growth and development.
3. *Nutritional Needs.* Requirements for specific nutrients do not appear to be different for diabetics than for nondiabetics. Therefore, the Recommended Dietary Allowance (RDA) and the *basic food groups* apply and should be used for planning and evaluation of diabetic diets. It has become evident through research that restriction of total carbohydrate to 40% or so of calories does not produce better diabetic control than diets higher in carbohydrate. In addition, when more carbohydrate is included, fat content can be lower. Diets lower in fat are particularly appropriate for the diabetic since degenerative vascular changes take place more rapidly than they do in the nondiabetic. The advice given in the *Dietary Guidelines for Americans* is especially helpful for diabetics.

4. *Meal Patterns.* Food, insulin, oral hypoglycenic agents, and exercise influence blood sugar concentration. These three influences need to be considered in various ways in the treatment of diabetics. When insulin therapy is used, the activity curve of the insulin determines the times of the day when needs for food are greatest. Exercise reduces insulin need and increases need for food. Usually a regular pattern for taking insulin injections, meals and snacks, and exercise can be worked out so that both hyperglycemia and hypoglycemia can be minimized. This is more important for the insulin dependent diabetic than for the diabetic not requiring insulin therapy.

5. *The Exchange Diet.* The Exchange Lists for Meal Planning were prepared by the American Dietetic Association (ADA) and the American Diabetes Association. The diet planning is based on the grouping of food into six categories. Foods in each group have comparable values; thus a food within a group may be exchanged or substituted for another in the same group. Included are eight meal patterns ranging from 1000 to 2800 calories. These are only suggested plans since the emphasis is on individualization as noted in Item 1.

6. *Measuring Food.* Food should be measured with standard measuring equipment (8 ounce cup, measuring spoons, small food scale, ruler) until the amounts can be estimated accurately. Checks should be made from time to time to make certain that measurements are accurate. Foods are measured after they are cooked. All measurements are level.

7. *Special Foods.* Special foods are not necessary. They are expensive and descriptions on foods labeled "dietetic" or "diabetic" are often misleading. If these products are used, it is necessary to compare calorie values with equal-sized portions of the usual product, because very often, even though sugar is omitted, enough fat, flour, nonfat milk solids, and other ingredients have been added to make the special product almost equal in calorie value to its ordinary counterpart. Since foods prepared for general meals should follow the principles of low fat, low sugar, low salt, and high fiber, the majority of these foods can be used for the diabetic also. If canned fruit packed in its own juice is used, the juice should not be given unless it is counted as another fruit exchange.

Composition of the Diabetic/Calorie-controlled Diet

Food Exchanges

Food	List	Amount	Weight	C^a	P^b	F^c	Cal
					(g)		
Starch/Bread	1	varies	–	15	3	tr	80
Meat	2	1 oz	30	–	7	5	75
Vegetable	3	1/2 cup	100	5	2	–	25
Fruit	4	varies	–	15	–	–	60
Milk (skim)	5	1 cup	240	12	8	tr	90
Fat	6	1 tsp	5	–	–	5	45

[a]Carbohydrate
[b]Protein
[c]Fat

Liquid and Clear Liquid Substitutions for a Diabetic Diet

When a diabetic patient cannot eat solid food it may be necessary to substitute liquid and/or clear liquid foods. The physician will often suggest the use of sweetened liquids to contribute toward meeting energy needs. The following table shows calorie and carbohydrate values for selected foods from the Liquid Diet.

Food	Amount	Carbohydrate	Calories
		(g)	
Carbonated beverages (swt)			
cola types	1 cup	24	95
ginger ale	1 cup	18	70
Cereal gruel (1/4 cup cereal, 1/4 cup milk)	1/2 cup	8	65
Creamed soup	1 cup	10	135
Custard, soft	1/2 cup	18	160
Eggnog	1 cup	20	230
Flavored gelatin	1/2 cup	17	70
Ice cream	1/2 cup	15	150
Ice milk	1/2 cup	20	145
Sherbet	1/2 cup	30	130
Sugar	1 tbsp.	12	45

Items such as milk, nonfat dry milk, fruit juices, and vegetable oil could be selected from the regular exchange lists and be used alone or in combination with any of the above. If the patient's problem is strictly a mechanical one, blenderizing menu items from the regular diabetic diet may be the answer.

FOOD EXCHANGE LISTS

The exchange lists of foods are based upon the grouping of foods into six categories—starch/breads, meats, vegetables, fruits, milk, and fats. Foods within each group have comparable value. Exchange means that a food listed in a particular group may be substituted or exchanged for another included in the same group. For example: 1 orange = 1 fruit exchange; 1 slice whole-wheat bread = 1 starch/bread exchange.

The serving size is important. Remember that each serving is 1 exchange. If the serving is doubled it equals 2 exchanges; 2 slices whole-wheat bread = 2 starch/bread exchanges. As stated, foods within each list may be exchanged for one another. For example:

1 starch/bread exchange = 1 slice bread

or

1 small potato

or

1/2 cup cooked cereal

The diet plan worked out by the dietitian for use with this food exchange list should be followed. Include the number of exchanges allowed from each food group every day, as suggested on the diet.

USING THE EXCHANGE LISTS IN MEAL PLANNING

An individualized meal plan should be developed by a dietitian who will take into account the patient's food preferences and life-style as well as caloric and other nutritional requirements.

The exchange lists provide an easy way to plan sensible, interesting, and nutritionally balanced meals. Common foods, except very concentrated sweets, will be found in one of the six exchange lists.

The exchange values of mixed dishes, such as casseroles, stews, and soups, can be determined if the amounts of the foods contained are known. The dietitian can teach patients to do this.

Foods may be substituted or exchanged for one another only within each exchange list.

These foods should generally be avoided because they have too much concentrated sugar. Small amounts may be allowed with the guidance of the dietitian.

Cakes	Jam
Candy	Jelly
Chewing gum	Pies
Condensed milk	Soft drinks
Cookies	Sugar
Honey	Syrup

LIST 1. STARCH/BREAD EXCHANGES

The list shows the kinds and amounts of breads, cereals, crackers, dried beans, starchy vegetables, and prepared foods to use for one bread exchange. Whole-grain products are recommended. If you want to eat a starch food that is not in the list, the general rule is that:

>   −1/2 cup of cereal, grain, or pasta is one serving
>   −1 ounce of a bread product is one serving

A dietitian can help you be more exact.

One starch/bread exchange contains:

Carbohydrate	15 g
Protein	3 g
Fat	trace
Calories	80

CEREALS/GRAINS/PASTA

Bran cereals, concentrated	1/3 cup
Bran cereals, flaked (such as Bran Buds, All Bran)	1/2 cup
Bulgur (cooked)	1/2 cup
Cooked cereals	1/2 cup
Cornmeal (dry)	2 1/2 tablespoons
Grapenuts	3 tablespoons
Grits (cooked)	1/2 cup
Other ready-to-eat unsweetened cereals	3/4 cup
Pasta (cooked)	1/2 cup
Puffed cereal	1 1/2 cup
Rice, white or brown (cooked)	1/3 cup
Shredded wheat	1/2 cup
Wheat germ	3 tablespoons

DRIED BEANS/PEAS/LENTILS

Beans and peas (cooked) (such as kidney, white, split, blackeye)	1/3 cup
Lentils (cooked)	1/3 cup
Baked beans	1/4 cup

STARCHY VEGETABLES

Corn	1/2 cup
Corn on cob, 6 in. long	1
Lima beans	1/2 cup
Peas, green (canned or frozen)	1/2 cup
Plantain	1/2 cup
Potato, baked	1 small (3 ounces)
Potato, mashed	1/2 cup
Squash, winter (acorn, butternut)	3/4 cup
Yam, sweet potato, plain	1/3 cup

BREAD

Bagel	1/2 (1 ounce)
Bread sticks, crisp, 4 in. long × 1/2 in.	2 (2/3 ounce)
Croutons, low fat	1 cup
English muffin	1/2
Frankfurter or hamburger bun	1/2 (1 ounce)
Pita, 6 in. across	1/2
Plain roll, small	1 (1 ounce)
Raisin, unfrosted	1 slice (1 ounce)
Rye, pumpernickel	1 slice (1 ounce)
Tortilla, 6 in. across	1
White (including French, Italian)	1 slice (1 ounce)
Whole-wheat	1 slice (1 ounce)

CRACKERS/SNACKS

Animal crackers	8
Graham crackers, 2 1/2 in. square	3
Matzoth	3/4 ounce
Melba toast	5 slices
Oyster crackers	24
Popcorn (popped, no fat added)	3 cups
Pretzels	3/4 ounce
Rye crisp, 2 in. × 3 1/2 in.	4
Saltine-type crackers	6
Whole-wheat crackers, no fat added (crisp breads, such as Finn, Kavli, Wasa)	2–4 slices (3/4 ounce)

STARCH FOODS PREPARED WITH FAT
(count as 1 starch/bread serving, plus 1 fat serving)

Biscuit, 2 1/2 in. across	1
Chow mein noodles	1/2 cup
Corn bread, 2 in. cube	1 (2 ounces)
Cracker, round butter-type	6
French fried potatoes, (2 in to 3 1/2 in. long)	10 (1 1/2 ounces)
Muffin, plain, small	1
Pancake, 4 in. across	2
Stuffing, bread (prepared)	1/4 cup
Taco shell, 6 in. across	2
Waffle, 4 1/2 in. square	1
Whole-wheat crackers, fat added (such as Triscuits)	4–6 (1 ounce)

LIST 2. MEAT EXCHANGES

Each serving of meat and substitutes on this list contains about 7 g of protein. The amount of fat and number of calories vary, depending on the kind of meat or substitute chosen. This list is divided into three parts based on the amount of fat and calories: lean meat, medium-fat meat, and high-fat meat.

LEAN MEAT AND SUBSTITUTES

One lean meat exchange contains:

Carbohydrate	0
Protein	7 g
Fat	3 g
Calories	55

Beef: USDA Good or Choice grades of lean beef, such as round steak, sirloin, and flank steak; tenderloin; and chipped beef — 1 ounce

Pork: Lean pork, such as fresh ham; canned, cured, or boiled ham; Canadian bacon; tenderloin — 1 ounce

Veal: All cuts are lean except for veal cutlets (ground or cubed); examples of lean veal are chops and roasts — 1 ounce

Poultry:	Chicken, turkey, Cornish hen (without skin)	1 ounce

Fish:	All fresh and frozen fish	1 ounce
	Crab, lobster, scallops, shrimp, clams (fresh or canned in water)	2 ounces
	Oysters	6 medium
	Tuna (canned in water)	1/4 cup
	Herring (uncreamed or smoked)	1 ounce
	Sardines (canned)	2 medium

Wild Game:	Venison, rabbit, squirrel	1 ounce
	Pheasant, duck, goose (without skin)	1 ounce

Cheese:	Any cottage cheese	1/4 cup
	Grated Parmesan	2 tablespoons
	Diet cheeses (with less than 55 calories per oz)	1 ounce

Other:	95% fat-free luncheon meat	1 ounce
	Egg whites	3 whites
	Egg substitutes with less than 55 calories per 1/4 cup	1/4 cup

MEDIUM-FAT MEAT AND SUBSTITUTES

One medium-fat meat exchange contains:

Carbohydrate	0
Protein	7 g
Fat	5 g
Calories	75

Beef:	Most beef products fall into this category; examples are all ground beef, roast (rib, chuck, rump), steak (cubed, Porterhouse, T-bone), and meatloaf.	1 ounce

Pork:	Most pork products fall into this category; examples are chops, loin roast, Boston butt, cutlets.	1 ounce

Lamb:	Most lamb products fall into this category; examples are chops, leg, and roast	1 ounce

Veal:	Cutlet (ground or cubed, unbreaded)	1 ounce
Poultry:	Chicken (with skin), domestic duck or goose (well drained of fat), ground turkey	1 ounce
Fish:	Tuna (canned in oil and drained)	1/4 cup
	Salmon (canned)	1/4 cup
Cheese:	Skim or part-skim milk cheeses such as:	
	Ricotta	1/4 cup
	Mozzarella	1 ounce
	Diet cheeses (with 56–80 calories per ounce)	1/4 cup
Other:	86% fat-free luncheon meat	1 ounce
	Egg (high in cholesterol, limit to 3 per week)	1
	Egg substitutes with 56–80 calories per 1/4 cup	1/4 cup
	Tofu (2 1/2 in. × 2 3/4 in. × 1 in.)	4 ounces
	Liver, heart, kidney, sweetbreads (high in cholesterol)	1 ounce

HIGH-FAT MEAT AND SUBSTITUTES

One high-fat meat exchange contains:

Carbohydrate	0	
Protein	7 g	
Fat	8 g	
Calories	100	

Remember, these items are high in saturated fat, cholesterol, and calories, and should be used minimally.

Beef:	Most USDA Prime cuts of beef, such as ribs, corned beef	1 ounce
Pork:	Spareribs, ground pork, pork sausage (patty or link)	1 ounce
Lamb:	Patties (ground lamb)	1 ounce
Fish:	Any fried fish product	1 ounce

Cheese: All regular cheeses, such as American,   1 ounce
            blue, cheddar, Monterey, Swiss

Other: Luncheon meat, such as bologna,   1 ounce
            salami, pimento loaf
            Sausage, such as Polish, Italian   1 ounce
            Knockwurst, smoked   1 ounce
            Bratwurst   1 ounce
            Frankfurter (turkey or chicken)   1 frank
                                                      (10/pound)

            Peanut butter (contains unsaturated   1 tablespoon
            fat)

Count as one high-fat meat plus one fat exchange:
            Frankfurter (beef, pork, or   1 frank
            combination)   (10/pound)

LIST 3. VEGETABLE EXCHANGES

Vegetables are good source of vitamins and minerals. Fresh and frozen vegetables have more vitamins and less added salt. Rinsing canned vegetables will remove much of the salt.

Unless otherwise noted, the serving size for vegetables (one vegetable exchange) is:

−1/2 cup of cooked vegetables or vegetable juice
−1 cup of raw vegetables

One vegetable exchange contains:

Carbohydrate	5 g
Protein	2 g
Fat	0
Calories	25

Artichoke (1/2 medium)   Mushrooms, cooked
Asparagus   Okra
Beans (green, wax, Italian)   Onions
Bean sprouts   Pea pods
Beets   Peppers (green)
Broccoli   Rutabaga
Brussels sprouts   Sauerkraut
Cabbage, cooked   Spinach, cooked

Carrots	Summer squash (crookneck)
Cauliflower	Tomato/vegetable juice
Eggplant	Turnips
Greens (collard, mustard, turnip)	Water chestnuts
Kohlrabi	Zucchini, cooked
Leeks	

Starchy vegetables such as corn, peas, and potatoes are found on the Starch/Bread list.

For free vegetables, see Free Foods in this section (following List 6).

LIST 4. FRUIT EXCHANGES

The carbohydrate and calorie content for a fruit serving are based on the usual serving of the most commonly eaten fruits. Use fresh fruits or fruits frozen or canned without sugar added. Whole fruit is more filling than fruit juice and may be a better choice for those who are trying to lose weight. Unless otherwise noted, the serving size for one fruit serving is:

    −1/2 cup of fresh fruit or fruit juice
    −1/4 cup of dried fruit

One fruit exchange contains:

	Carbohydrate	15 g
	Protein	0
	Fat	0
	Calories	60

FRESH, FROZEN, AND UNSWEETENED CANNED FRUIT

Apple (raw, 2 in. across)	1
Applesauce (unsweetened)	1/2 cup
Apricots (medium, raw)	4
Apricots (canned)	1/2 cup or 4 halves
Banana (9 in. long)	1/2
Blackberries (raw)	3/4 cup
Blueberries (raw)	3/4 cup
Cantaloupe (5 in. across)	1/3
(cubes)	1 cup
Cherries (large, raw)	12
Cherries (canned)	1/2 cup
Figs (raw, 2 in. across)	2

Fruit cocktail (canned)	1/2 cup
Grapefruit (medium)	1/2
Grapefruit (segments)	3/4 cup
Grapes (small)	15
Honeydew melon (medium)	1/8
(cubes)	1 cup
Kiwi (large)	1
Mandarin oranges	3/4 cup
Mango (small)	1/2
Nectarine (1 1/2 in across)	1
Orange (2 1/2 in. across)	1
Papaya	1 cup
Peach (2 3/4 in. across)	1 peach or 3/4 cup
Peaches (canned)	1/2 cup or 2 halves
Pear	1/2 large or 1 small
Pears (canned)	1/2 cup or 2 halves
Persimmon (medium, native)	2
Pineapple (raw)	3/4 cup
Pineapple (canned)	1/3 cup
Plum (raw, 2 in. across)	2
Pomegranate	1/2
Raspberries (raw)	1 cup
Strawberries (raw, whole)	1 1/4 cup
Tangerine (2 1/2 in. across)	2
Watermelon (cubes)	1 1/4 cup

DRIED FRUIT

Apples	4 rings
Apricots	7 halves
Dates	2 1/2 medium
Figs	1 1/2
Prunes	3 medium
Raisins	2 tablespoons

FRUIT JUICE

Apple juice/cider	1/2 cup
Cranberry juice cocktail	1/3 cup
Grapefruit juice	1/2 cup
Grape juice	1/3 cup
Orange juice	1/2 cup
Pineapple juice	1/2 cup
Prune juice	1/3 cup

LIST 5. MILK EXCHANGES

Milk is the body's main source of calcium, the mineral needed for growth and repair of bones. Yogurt is also a good source of calcium.

Each serving of milk or milk products on this list contains the same amount of carbohydrate and protein. The amount of fat in milk, as measured by percentage (%) of butterfat, varies. This causes the difference in calories among the three types.

One serving (one milk exchange) of each of these includes:

	Carbohydrate (g)	Protein (g)	Fat (g)	Calories
Skim/Very Lowfat	12	8	trace	90
Lowfat	12	8	5	120
Whole	12	8	8	150

SKIM AND VERY LOWFAT MILK
Skim milk	1 cup
1/2% milk	1 cup
1% milk	1 cup
Lowfat buttermilk	1 cup
Evaporated skim milk	1/2 cup
Dry nonfat milk	1/3 cup
Plain nonfat yogurt	8 ounces

LOWFAT MILK
2% milk	1 cup
Plain lowfat yogurt (with added nonfat milk solids)	8 ounces

WHOLE MILK
The whole milk group has much more fat per serving than the skim and lowfat groups. Whole milk has more than 3 1/4% butterfat. Limit choices from the whole milk group as much as possible.

Whole milk	1 cup
Evaporated whole milk	1/2 cup
Whole plain yogurt	8 ounces

LIST 6. FAT EXCHANGES

The foods on the fat list contain mostly fat, although some items may also contain a small amount of protein. All fats are high in calories and should be carefully measured. Everyone should modify fat intake by eating unsaturated fats instead of saturated fats.

One fat exchange contains:		
	Carbohydrate	0
	Protein	0
	Fat	5 g
	Calories	45

UNSATURATED FATS

Avocado (medium)	1/8
Margarine	1 teaspoon
Margarine, diet	1 tablespoon
Mayonnaise	1 teaspoon
Mayonnaise, reduced-calorie	1 tablespoon
Nuts and Seeds:	
Almonds, dry roasted (whole)	6
Cashews, dry roasted	1 tablespoon
Pecans (whole)	2
Peanuts	20 small or 10 large
Walnuts (whole)	2
Other nuts	1 tablespoon
Seeds, pine nuts, sunflower (without shells)	1 tablespoon
Pumpkin seeds	2 teaspoons
Oil (corn, cottonseed, safflower, soybean, sunflower, olive, peanut)	1 teaspoon
Olives	10 small or 5 large
Salad dressing, mayonnaise-type	2 teaspoons
Salad dressing, mayonnaise-type, reduced-calorie	1 tablespoon
Salad dressing (all varieties)	1 tablespoon
Salad dressing, reduced-calorie	2 tablespoon

(two tablespoons of low-calorie salad dressing is a free food)

SATURATED FATS

Butter	1 teaspoon
Bacon	1 slice
Chitterlings	1/2 ounce

Coconut, shredded	2 tablespoons
Coffee whitener, liquid	2 tablespoons
Coffee whitener, powder	4 teaspoons
Cream (light, coffee, table)	2 tablespoons
Cream, sour	2 tablespoons
Cream (heavy, whipping)	1 tablespoon
Cream cheese	1 tablespoon
Salt pork	1/4 ounce

FREE FOODS

Free foods or drinks contain less than 20 calories per serving. These may be used in unlimited amounts if no serving size is specified (unless restricted for some other reason).

DRINKS
Bouillon or broth,
  without fat
Bouillon, low-sodium
Carbonated drinks,
  sugar-free
Carbonated water
Club soda
Cocoa powder,
  unsweetened (1 tablespoon)
Coffee/Tea
Drink mixes, sugar-free
Tonic water, sugar-free

FRUIT
Cranberries, unsweetened
  (1/2 cup)
Rhubarb, unsweetened
  (1/2 cup)

CONDIMENTS
Catsup (1 tablespoon)
Horseradish
Mustard

Pickles, dill,
  unsweetened
Salad dressing, low-calorie
  (2 tablespoons)
Taco sauce (1 tablespoon)
Vinegar

VEGETABLES
(Raw, 1 cup)
Cabbage
Celery
Chinese cabbage
Cucumber
Green onion
Hot peppers
Mushrooms
Radishes
Zucchini

SALAD GREENS
Endive
Escarole
Lettuce
Romaine
Spinach

SWEET SUBSTITUTES

Candy, hard, sugar-free
Gelatin, sugar-free
Gum, sugar-free
Jam/Jelly, sugar-free
  (2 teaspoons)

Pancake syrup, sugar-free
  (1–2 tablespoons)
Sugar substitutes
  (saccharin, aspartame)
Whipped topping
  (2 tablespoons)

Spices and seasonings can make foods taste better. Use sugar-free, fat-free spices and seasonings as desired. Some seasonings are very high in sodium. Their use is limited in sodium-restricted diets.

FOODS FOR OCCASIONAL USE

Moderate amounts of some foods can be used in a meal plan, in spite of their sugar or fat content, as long as blood-glucose control is maintained. The following is a list of some of these foods with their average exchange values. Because they are sources of concentrated carbohydrates (sugars), portion sizes are very small. Check with a dietitian for advice on their use in a meal plan.

Food	Amount	Exchanges
Angel food cake	1/12 cake	2 starch
Cake, no icing	1/12 cake, or a 3 in. square	2 starch, 2 fat
Cookies	2 small (1 3/4 in. across)	1 starch, 1 fat
Frozen fruit yogurt	1/3 cup	1 starch
Gingersnaps	3	1 starch
Granola	1/4 cup	1 starch, 1 fat
Granola bars	1 small	1 starch, 1 fat
Ice cream, any flavor	1/2 cup	1 starch, 2 fat
Ice milk, any flavor	1/2 cup	1 starch, 1 fat
Sherbet, any flavor	1/4 cup	1 starch
Snack chips, all varieties	1 ounce	1 starch, 2 fat
Vanilla wafers	6 small	1 starch, 1 fat

Source: The Exchange Lists are the basis of a meal planning system designed by a committee of the American Diabetes Association and the American Dietetic Association. While designed primarily for people with diabetes and others who must follow special diets, the Exchange Lists are based on principles of good nutrition that apply to everyone. © 1986 American Diabetes Association, Inc., American Dietetic Association.

CALORIE-CONTROLLED DIETS

Use: The Calorie-controlled Diets are prescribed for weight reduction and weight control.

Adequacy: With the exception of the 1000 Calorie Diet, the Calorie-controlled Diets include foods in amounts that will provide the quantities of nutrients (except iron for females) recommended by the NRC for the average adult. The 1000 Calorie Diet may be marginal in meeting these recommendations.

Diet Principles:
1. The Calorie-controlled Diets use the diabetic patterns, both in choice and distribution of carbohydrate, protein, and fat.
2. The Calorie-controlled Diets are planned to permit an individual to lose weight and still maintain heath. This requires an adequate intake of protein, minerals, and vitamins. It is important, therefore, that an individual eat all the food allowed on the diet.
3. After a period of weight loss on a reduction diet, an individual may remain the same weight for one, two, or even three weeks. Weight loss will resume, however, if the diet is continued.
4. The suggested menu plan may be modified to meet individual desires. For example, if an individual would like a midafternoon or evening snack, s/he may reserve some food from the previous meal for that purpose, or s/he may divide the food for the day into five small meals instead of the suggested three.

MEAL PATTERNS FOR DIABETIC/CALORIE-CONTROLLED DIETS

CALORIE LEVEL	1000	1200	1500	1800	2000	2200	2800	1800[a]
TOTAL FOOD EXCHANGES								
Starch/Bread	3	4	6	7	8	10	12	7
Meat	4	5	5	6	7	7	9	6
Vegetable	2	2	2	2	3	3	4	2
Fruit	3	3	3	4	4	4	6	3
Milk, skim	2	2	2	3	3	3	4	4
Fat	2	3	5	5	6	7	8	5
SAMPLE MEAL PATTERN								
BREAKFAST								
Starch/Bread	1	1	1	2	3	3	4	2
Meat	0	0	0	0	0	0	0	0
Fruit	1	1	1	1	1	1	2	1
Milk, skim	½	½	½	1	1	1	1	1
Fat	½	1	1	1	2	2	2	1
LUNCH								
Starch/Bread	½	1	2	2	2	3	3	2
Meat	2	2	2	3	3	3	4	3
Vegetable, raw				----------as desired----------				
Vegetable	1	1	1	1	1	1	2	1
Fruit	1	1	1	1	1	1	1	1
Milk, skim	½	½	½	1	1	1	1	1
Fat	½	1	2	2	2	2	2	2

MEAL PATTERNS FOR DIABETIC/CALORIE-CONTROLLED DIETS (continued)

CALORIE LEVEL	1000	1200	1500	1800	2000	2200	2800	1800*
DINNER								
Starch/Bread	1	1	2	2	2	2	3	2
Meat	2	3	3	3	3	3	4	3
Vegetable, raw				--------as desired--------				
Vegetable	1	1	1	1	2	2	2	1
Fruit	1	1	1	1	1	1	2	1
Milk, skim	½	½	½	½	½	½	1	1
Fat	1	1	2	2	2	3	4	2
SNACK								
Starch/Bread	½	1	1	1	1	2	2	1
Meat	0	0	0	0	1	1	1	0
Fruit	0	0	0	1	1	1	1	0
Milk, skim	½	½	½	½	½	½	1	1
Fat	0	0	0	0	0	0	0	0
APPROXIMATE COMPOSITION								
CALORIES	1039	1238	1490	1793	2020	2227	2817	1822
CARBOHYDRATE (g)	124	139	169	211	231	261	338	208
(% Calories)	(48)	(45)	(45)	(47)	(46)	(47)	(48)	(46)
PROTEIN (g)	57	67	73	91	103	109	139	99
(% Calories)	(22)	(22)	(20)	(20)	(20)	(20)	(20)	(22)
FAT (g)[b]	35	46	58	65	76	83	101	66
(% Calories)	(30)	(33)	(35)	(33)	(34)	(33)	(32)	(32)

[a]1800 calorie diet that includes 4 cups milk is included for an adolescent or a pregnant woman.
[b]Calculations based on 1 g fat for each starch/bread and skim milk exchange.

SUGGESTED MENUS FOR DIABETIC CALORIE-CONTROLLED DIETS

1000 CALORIE DIET

Carbohydrate	124 g	(48% calories)
Protein	57 g	(22% calories)
Fat	35 g	(30% calories)

MEAL PATTERN			SAMPLE MENU
			Breakfast
1	Fruit	1/2 cup	Orange juice
1	Starch/Bread	1 slice	Whole-grain toast
1/2	Fat	1/2 teaspoon	Margarine or butter
1/2	Skim milk	1/2 cup	Skim milk
			Lunch
1/2	Starch/Bread	1/2 slice	Whole-grain bread for open-face sandwich with
2	Meat	2 ounces	Sliced lean roast beef
	Raw vegetable		Lettuce leaf, tomato slice for sandwich
1/2	Fat	1/2 teaspoon	Reduced fat mayonnaise for sandwich
1	Vegetable	1/2 cup	Steamed carrots
1	Fruit	1 medium	Apple
1/2	Skim milk	1/2 cup	Skim milk
			Dinner
2	Meat	2 ounces	Baked fish with lemon and parsley
1	Starch/Bread	1/3 cup	Brown rice
1	Vegetable	1/2 cup	Steamed broccoli
	Raw vegetable		Tossed fresh vegetable salad
1	Fat	1 teaspoon	Oil for vinegar and oil dressing
1	Fruit	1/3 cup	Water packed pineapple chunks
1/2	Skim milk	1/2 cup	Skim milk
			Snack
1/2	Skim milk	1/2 cup	Skim milk
1/2	Starch/Bread	1 1/2 squares	Graham crackers

1200 CALORIE DIET

Carbohydrate	139 g	(45% calories)
Protein	67 g	(22% calories)
Fat	46 g	(33% calories)

MEAL PATTERN   SAMPLE MENU

Breakfast

1	Fruit	1/2	cup	Orange juice
1	Starch/Bread	1	slice	Whole-grain toast with
1	Fat	1	teaspoon	Margarine or butter
1/2	Skim milk	1/2	cup	Skim milk

Lunch

1	Starch/Bread	1	slice	Whole-grain bread for sandwich with
2	Meat	2	ounces	Sliced lean roast beef
	Raw vegetable			Lettuce leaf, tomato slice for sandwich
1	Fat	1	teaspoon	Mayonnaise for sandwich
1	Vegetable	1/2	cup	Steamed carrots
1	Fruit	1	medium	Apple
1/2	Skim milk	1/2	cup	Skim milk

Dinner

3	Meat	3	ounces	Baked fish with lemon and parsley
1	Starch/Bread	1/3	cup	Brown rice
1	Vegetable	1/2	cup	Steamed broccoli
	Raw vegetable			Tossed fresh vegetable salad
1	Fat	1	teaspoon	Oil for vinegar and oil dressing
1	Fruit	1/3	cup	Water packed pineapple chunks
1/2	Skim milk	1/2	cup	Skim milk

Snack

1/2	Skim milk	1/2	cup	Skim milk
1	Starch/Bread	3	squares	Graham crackers

1500 CALORIE DIET

Carbohydrate	169 g	(45% calories)
Protein	73 g	(20% calories)
Fat	58 g	(35% calories)

MEAL PATTERN			SAMPLE MENU

Breakfast

1	Fruit	1/2	cup	Orange juice
1	Starch/Bread	1	slice	Whole-grain toast with
1	Fat	1	teaspoon	Margarine or butter
1/2	Skim milk	1/2	cup	Skim milk

Lunch

2	Starch/Bread	2	slices	Whole-grain bread for sandwich with
2	Meat	2	ounces	Sliced lean roast beef
	Raw vegetable			Lettuce leaf, tomato slice for sandwich
2	Fat	2	teaspoons	Mayonnaise for sandwich
1	Vegetable	1/2	cup	Steamed carrots
1	Fruit	1	medium	Apple
1/2	Skim milk	1/2	cup	Skim milk

Dinner

3	Meat	3	ounces	Baked fish with lemon and parsley
1	Starch/Bread	1/3	cup	Brown rice
1	Vegetable	1/2	cup	Steamed broccoli
	Raw vegetable			Tossed fresh vegetable salad
1	Fat	1	teaspoon	Oil for vinegar and oil dressing
1	Starch/Bread	1		Whole-grain dinner roll
1	Fat	1	teaspoon	Margarine or butter
1	Fruit	1/3	cup	Water packed pineapple chunks
1/2	Skim milk	1/2	cup	Skim milk

Snack

1/2	Skim milk	1/2	cup	Skim milk
1	Starch/Bread	3	squares	Graham crackers

1800 CALORIE DIET

Carbohydrate	211 g	(47% calories)
Protein	91 g	(20% calories)
Fat	65 g	(33% calories)

MEAL PATTERN   SAMPLE MENU

Breakfast

1	Fruit	1/2	cup	Orange juice
2	Starch/Bread	1/2	cup	Oatmeal
		1	slice	Whole-grain toast with
1	Fat	1	teaspoon	Margarine or butter
1	Skim milk	1	cup	Skim milk

Lunch

2	Starch/Bread	2	slices	Whole-grain bread for sandwich with
3	Meat	3	ounces	Sliced lean roast beef
	Raw vegetables			Lettuce leaf, tomato slice for sandwich
2	Fat	2	teaspoons	Mayonnaise for sandwich
1	Vegetable	1/2	cup	Steamed carrots
1	Fruit	1	medium	Apple
1	Skim milk	1	cup	Skim milk

Dinner

3	Meat	3	ounces	Baked fish with lemon and parsley
1	Starch/Bread	1/3	cup	Brown rice
1	Vegetable	1/2	cup	Steamed broccoli
	Raw vegetable			Tossed fresh vegetable salad
1	Fat	1	teaspoon	Oil for vinegar and oil dressing
1	Starch/Bread	1		Whole-grain dinner roll
1	Fat	1	teaspoon	Margarine or butter
1	Fruit	1/3	cup	Water packed pineapple chunks
1/2	Skim milk	1/2	cup	Skim milk

Snack

1/2	Skim milk	1/2	cup	Skim milk
1	Starch/Bread	2	squares	Rye Krisp
1	Fruit	1	small	Pear

2000 CALORIE DIET

Carbohydrate	231 g	(46% calories)
Protein	103 g	(20% calories)
Fat	76 g	(34% calories)

MEAL PATTERN			SAMPLE MENU

Breakfast

1	Fruit	1/2	cup	Orange juice
1	Starch/Bread	1/2	cup	Oatmeal
2	Starch/Bread	2	slices	Whole-grain toast with
2	Fat	2	teaspoons	Margarine or butter
1	Skim milk	1	cup	Skim milk

Lunch

2	Starch/Bread	2	slices	Whole-grain bread for sandwich with
3	Meat	3	ounces	Sliced lean roast beef
	Raw vegetables			Lettuce leaf, tomato slice for sandwich
2	Fat	2	teaspoons	Mayonnaise for sandwich
1	Vegetable	1/2	cup	Steamed carrots
1	Fruit	1	medium	Apple
1	Skim milk	1	cup	Skim milk

Dinner

3	Meat	3	ounces	Baked fish with lemon and parsley
1	Starch/Bread	1/3	cup	Brown rice
2	Vegetable	1	cup	Steamed broccoli
	Raw vegetable			Tossed fresh vegetable salad
1	Fat	1	teaspoon	Oil for vinegar and oil dressing
1	Starch/Bread	1		Whole-grain dinner roll
1	Fat	1	teaspoon	Margarine or butter
1	Fruit	1/3	cup	Water packed pineapple chunks
1/2	Skim milk	1/2	cup	Skim milk

Snack

1/2	Skim milk	1/2	cup	Skim milk
1	Starch/Bread	2	squares	Rye Krisp
1	Meat	1/4	cup	2% cottage cheese
1	Fruit	1	small	Pear

2200 CALORIE DIET

Carbohydrate	261 g	(47% calories)
Protein	109 g	(20% calories)
Fat	83 g	(33% calories)

MEAL PATTERN   SAMPLE MENU

Breakfast

1	Fruit	1/2	cup	Orange juice
1	Starch/Bread	1/2	cup	Oatmeal
2	Starch/Bread	2	slices	Whole-grain toast with
2	Fat	2	teaspoons	Margarine or butter
1	Skim milk	1	cup	Skim milk

Lunch

2	Starch/Bread	2	slices	Whole-grain bread for sandwich with
3	Meat	3	ounces	Sliced lean roast beef
	Raw vegetables			Lettuce leaf, tomato slice for sandwich
2	Fat	2	teaspoons	Mayonnaise for sandwich
1	Vegetable	1/2	cup	Steamed carrots
1	Fruit	1	medium	Apple
1	Skim milk	1	cup	Skim milk
1	Starch/Bread	1/4	cup	Sherbert

Dinner

3	Meat	3	ounces	Baked fish with lemon and parsley
1	Starch/Bread	1/3	cup	Brown rice
2	Vegetable	1	cup	Steamed broccoli
	Raw vegetable			Tossed fresh vegetable salad
1	Fat	1	teaspoon	Oil for vinegar and oil dressing
1	Starch/Bread	1		Whole-grain dinner roll
2	Fat	2	teaspoons	Margarine or butter
1	Fruit	1/3	cup	Water packed pineapple chunks
1/2	Skim milk	1/2	cup	Skim milk

Snack

1/2	Skim milk	1/2	cup	Skim milk
2	Starch/Bread	6	squares	Graham crackers
1	Meat	1	tablespoon	Peanut butter
1	Fruit	1	small	Pear

2800 CALORIE DIET

Carbohydrate	338 g	(48% calories)
Protein	139 g	(20% calories)
Fat	101 g	(32% calories)

MEAL PATTERN   SAMPLE MENU

Breakfast

1	Fruit	1/2	cup	Orange juice
2	Starch/Bread	1	cup	Oatmeal
1	Fruit	2	tablespoons	Raisins
2	Starch/Bread	2	slices	Whole-grain toast with
2	Fat	2	teaspoons	Margarine or butter
1	Skim milk	1	cup	Skim milk

Lunch

2	Starch/Bread	2	slices	Whole-grain bread for sandwich with
4	Meat	4	ounces	Sliced lean roast beef
	Raw vegetables			Lettuce leaf, tomato slice for sandwich
2	Fat	2	teaspoons	Mayonnaise for sandwich
2	Vegetable	1	cup	Steamed carrots
1	Fruit	1	medium	Apple
1	Skim milk	1	cup	Skim milk
1	Starch/Bread	1/4	cup	Sherbet

Dinner

4	Meat	4	ounces	Baked fish with lemon and parsley
1	Starch/Bread	1/3	cup	Brown rice
2	Vegetable	1	cup	Steamed broccoli
	Raw vegetable			Tossed fresh vegetable salad
2	Fat	2	teaspoons	Oil for vinegar and oil dressing
2	Starch/Bread	2		Whole-grain dinner rolls
2	Fat	2	teaspoons	Margarine or butter
2	Fruit	2/3	cup	Water packed pineapple chunks
1	Skim milk	1	cup	Skim milk

Snack

1	Skim milk	1	cup	Skim milk
2	Starch/Bread	6	squares	Graham crackers
1	Meat	1 tablespoon		Peanut butter
1	Fruit	1	small	Pear

1800 CALORIE DIET FOR ADOLESCENT, OR PREGNANT WOMAN[*]

Carbohydrate	208 g	(46% calories)
Protein	99 g	(22% calories)
Fat	66 g	(32% calories)

MEAL PATTERN			SAMPLE MENU
		Breakfast	
1	Fruit	1/2 cup	Orange juice
1	Starch/Bread	1/2 cup	Oatmeal
1	Starch/Bread	1 slice	Whole-grain toast with
1	Fat	1 teaspoon	Margarine or butter
1	Skim milk	1 cup	Skim milk
		Lunch	
2	Starch/Bread	2 slices	Whole-grain bread for sandwich with
3	Meat	3 ounces	Sliced lean roast beef
	Raw vegetable		Lettuce leaf, tomato slice for sandwich
2	Fat	2 teaspoons	Mayonnaise for sandwich
1	Vegetable	1/2 cup	Steamed carrots
1	Fruit	1 medium	Apple
1	Skim milk	1 cup	Skim milk
		Dinner	
3	Meat	3 ounces	Baked fish with lemon and parsley
1	Starch/Bread	1/3 cup	Brown rice
1	Vegetable	1/2 cup	Steamed broccoli
	Raw vegetable		Tossed fresh vegetable salad
1	Fat	1 teaspoon	Oil for vinegar and oil dressing
1	Starch/Bread	1	Whole-grain dinner roll
1	Fat	1 teaspoon	Margarine or butter
1	Fruit	1/3 cup	Water packed pineapple chunks
1	Skim milk	1 cup	Skim milk
		Snack	
1	Skim milk	1 cup	Skim milk
1	Starch/Bread	3 squares	Graham crackers

---

[*]This pattern includes 4 cups milk.

Modified Diets

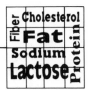

LOW FIBER, LOW RESIDUE DIET

Use: The Low Fiber, Low Residue Diet is designed for patients receiving radiation therapy on or near the intestine, in partial bowel obstruction, in acute gastroenteritis, and in postoperative anal or hemorrhoidal surgery.

Adequacy: The suggested food plan includes foods in amounts that will provide the quantities of nutrients (except iron for females) recommended by the NRC for the average adult, providing the individual can tolerate milk.

Diet Principles: The diet includes foods that will reduce (not eliminate) the residue in the colon. It is smooth in texture and is mechanically and chemically nonirritating.

FOOD FOR THE DAY	DESCRIPTION	
	Allowed	**Avoid**
MILK *limit to 2 cups*	All milk and milk drinks; yogurt. If an individual does not tolerate milk to drink, use in cooking or boil before serving.	Yogurt, if flavored with fruit containing small seeds; milk or yogurt in excess of 2 cups
MEAT and MEAT SUBSTITUTES *2 servings* *(4-6 ounces)*	Tender beef, chicken, fish, ham, lamb, liver, pork, turkey, veal; cottage cheese, cream cheese, mild natural, or processed cheese; eggs; smooth peanut butter, if tolerated	Unless tolerated: spicy meat, fish, poultry; strongly flavored cheeses
FRUITS *2-3 servings*	Any not listed to avoid	Prune juice; apples (fresh), bananas, most berries, currants, figs, oranges, pears (fresh), prunes
VEGETABLES *2-3 servings*	Any not listed to avoid; all vegetable juices	Cooked dried beans and legumes, corn, peas, spinach, potato skin, winter squash, artichoke

FOOD FOR THE DAY	DESCRIPTION	
	Allowed	**Avoid**
	Choices of fruits and vegetables should include a good source (or two fair sources) of vitamin C daily and a good source of vitamin A at least every other day	
BREADS, CEREALS, and GRAINS *4 or more servings*	Enriched white, wheat, rye bread without seeds; saltines, rusk, zwieback, Melba toast; enriched, cooked, refined cereals, such as farina, Cream of Wheat, cornmeal, Malt-o-Meal, strained oatmeal; dry cereals such as puffed rice, riceflakes, cornflakes; spaghetti, macaroni, noodles, or rice	Bread, crackers, or cereals containing whole grains, bran, or seeds; brown or wild rice
FATS *in moderate amounts*	Salad oils, fortified margarine, butter, cream, mayonnaise, mildly seasoned salad dressings; crisp bacon	Spicy salad dressings
FLUID *6-8 cups*	Water and other fluids, such as coffee, tea, fruit or vegetable juice, carbonated beverages	
OTHER	Homemade, strained soups made with thin cream sauce and allowed vegetables; clear broth soups	All others
	Plain puddings; plain ice cream; sherbet without fruit pulp; plain cakes and pies made from allowed foods; honey, syrups, hard candy	All desserts and candy containing coconut, nuts, seeds, or fruit; jams and preserves
	Mild catsup, mild spices, vinegar, white sauce in moderate amounts	Pepper, spicy catsup, chili sauce, nuts, olives, coconut, pickles, popcorn

Suggested Menu Plan for Low Fiber, Low Residue Diet
(Select from foods described)

Breakfast
Citrus fruit juice
Cereal with 1/2 cup milk and/or egg
Toast or bread with margarine or butter
Beverage

Lunch or Supper
Meat or substitute
Potato, pasta, or grain
Vegetable
Bread with margarine or butter
Fruit
1/2 cup milk

Dinner
Meat or substitute
Potato, pasta, or grain
Vegetable
Bread with margarine or butter
1 cup yogurt

LOW FAT DIET
(40-50 g fat)

Use: The Low Fat Diet may be prescribed to reduce the fat intake for patients with diseases of the gallbladder, liver, pancreas, or if disturbances in digestion and absorption of fat occur.

Adequacy: The suggested food plan includes foods in amounts that will provide the quantities of nutrients (except iron for females) recommended by the NRC for the average adult. Restriction of fat (the most concentrated source of calories) may result in a diet low in calories. When additional calories are needed, add them in the form of complex carbohydrate.

Diet Principles:
1. The diet is designed to limit the fat intake and to restrict the fats to those that are highly emulsified and readily digested. Fried foods and other foods that cause gastrointestinal tract distress in many individuals are limited or omitted.
2. This diet contains approximately 40–50 g of fat per day.
3. Foods may cause distress for reasons other than fat content. Tolerance varies greatly among people. If a food is tolerated, it may be allowed.

FOOD FOR THE DAY	DESCRIPTION	
	Allowed	**Avoid**
MILK *2 or more cups*	Skim milk, nonfat dry milk, buttermilk made from skim milk; yogurt	Cream, whole milk, 2% milk; ice cream, ice milk
EGGS *(if tolerated)* *(Limit to 1 yolk per day including cooking.)*	Poached, soft- or hard-cooked; scrambled without fat; egg white as desired	Fried eggs
MEAT and MEAT SUBSTITUTES *2 servings* *(total 4-5 ounces)*	Lean beef, pork, lamb, veal, poultry; lean fish, such as cod, flounder, haddock, bluefish, perch, bass, whitefish; lowfat cottage cheese, lowfat Monterey Jack, mozzarella made from skim milk, ricotta, farmer cheese made from skim milk	Luncheon meat, frankfurters, corned beef; smoked, spiced, processed meats or fish; fatty fish or fish packed in oil; all other cheese; peanut butter

FOOD FOR THE DAY	DESCRIPTION	
	Allowed	**Avoid**
FRUITS *2 or more servings*	Any fresh, frozen, dried, or canned fruits; fruit juice	Any fruit if not tolerated
VEGETABLES *2 or more servings* *(including potato)*	All fresh, frozen, or canned vegetables; vegetable juice	Any that may cause discomfort: cabbage family, onion, peppers, radishes
	White or sweet potato, yams. Any fat used must be taken from the fat allowance.	Fried potatoes, potato chips, creamed potatoes
	Choices of fruits and vegetables should include a good source (or two fair sources) of vitamin C daily and a good source of vitamin A at least every other day.	
BREADS, CEREALS, and GRAINS *4 or more servings*	Whole-grain or enriched breads, cereals, and grains; whole-grain or enriched macaroni, spaghetti, noodles, or rice	Hot breads, such as muffins, biscuits, rich rolls, sweet rolls, and doughnuts; party crackers; granola, 100% bran unless well tolerated
FATS *Limit to 1 tablespoon*	Butter, fortified margarine, or salad oil. Use on bread, salads, or in cooking.	
FLUID *6-8 cups*	Water and other fluids, such as coffee, tea, fruit or vegetable juice	

FOOD FOR THE DAY	DESCRIPTION	
	Allowed	**Avoid**
OTHER	Homemade soups made with fat-free broth or skim milk, with or without allowed vegetables	Commercial soups; soups prepared with cream or whole milk
	Gelatin desserts; angel food cake, vanilla wafers, arrowroot cookies; sherbet, puddings prepared with skim milk	Nuts, olives, chocolate, coconut, popcorn, candy containing nuts or fat
	Sugar, syrup, honey; plain jelly and jam; gumdrops and hard candy	
	All spices, seasonings, and flavorings in moderate amounts; cocoa powder	

Suggested Menu Plan for Low Fat Diet
(Select from foods described)

The carbohydrate, protein, fat and calories will vary depending upon whether the smaller or larger amounts of food are served. Fats are high in calories, and when fats are restricted calories are provided through foods high in carbohydrate.

Breakfast
Fruit or fruit juice
Cereal/egg
Whole-grain bread
Margarine or butter (1 teaspoon)*
Skim milk
Hot beverage

Lunch or Supper
Lean meat or substitute (2 ounces)
Vegetable
Whole-grain bread
Margarine or butter (1 teaspoon)*
Fruit
Skim milk

Dinner
Lean meat or substitute (2–3 ounces)
Potato, pasta, or grain
Vegetable
Whole-grain bread
Margarine or butter (1 teaspoon)*
Fruit
Skim milk

Snacks
Skim milk, fruits, crackers, fresh
  vegetables

---

*Use on bread or in cooking.

MODERATE CHOLESTEROL/FAT RESTRICTED DIET
(300 mg cholesterol, 30% of calories from fat)

Use: The Moderate Cholesterol/Fat Restricted Diet is prescribed in an effort to reduce the cholesterol and other fatty substances in the blood for the treatment of hyperlipidemia.

Adequacy: The suggested food plan includes foods in amounts that will provide the quantities of nutrients (except iron for females) recommended by the NRC for the average adult.

Diet Principles:
1. Dietary cholesterol is reduced to 300 mg or less per day.
2. A maximum of 30% of calories comes from fat.
3. The proportion of saturated fat is decreased. The ratio of polyunsaturated fat to saturated fat is increased.
4. Complex carbohydrates are increased to replace fat.
5. These diet suggestions may be liberalized for a geriatric patient.

FOOD FOR THE DAY	DESCRIPTION	
	Allowed	**Avoid**
MILK *2 or more cups*	Skim milk, nonfat dry milk, buttermilk made from skim milk; skim milk yogurt	Cream, whole milk, 2% milk; ice cream, ice milk
EGGS *(Limit yolks to 4 per week.)*	Poached, soft- or hard-cooked, scrambled without fat; egg white as desired; egg substitutes Count egg yolks used in cooking as well as those eaten as such.	Fried egg
MEAT and MEAT SUBSTITUTES *2 servings* *(total 4-5 ounces)*	Lean beef, pork, lamb, veal, poultry; lean fish, such as cod, flounder, haddock, bluefish, perch, bass, whitefish; low fat cottage cheese, low fat Monterey Jack, mozzarella made from skim milk, and ricotta; farmer cheese from skim milk	Fat beef, pork, lamb, and any visible fat on meat; bacon, salt pork, spareribs, frankfurters, sausage, cold cuts, canned meats; skin of chicken or turkey, duck, goose; fish roe, fish canned in oil; organ meats; cheese other than that allowed

FOOD FOR THE DAY	DESCRIPTION	
	Allowed	**Avoid**
FRUITS *2 or more servings*	Any fresh, frozen, dried, or canned fruits; fruit juice	Avocado
VEGETABLES *2 or more servings* *(including potato)*	All fresh, frozen, or canned vegetables; vegetable juice; white or sweet potato, yams. Any fat used must be taken from the fat allowance. Choices of fruits and vegetables should include a good source (or two fair sources) of vitamin C daily and a good source of vitamin A at least every other day.	
BREAD, CEREALS, and GRAINS *4 or more servings*	Whole-grain or enriched breads, cereals, and grains; Melba toast, matzo bread sticks, rye wafers, saltines, graham crackers, pretzels; hot bread, griddle cakes, waffles made with egg substitute or egg white and allowed fats	Commercial hot breads, doughnuts, sweet rolls; egg or cheese breads; party crackers
FATS *(Limit to 1 1/2-2* *tablespoons)*	See list of unsaturated fats on page 58.	Butter, ordinary margarine; ordinary solid shortening, lard, salt pork, chicken fat, coconut oil, chocolate
FLUID *6-8 cups*	Water and other fluids, such as coffee, tea, fruit or vegetable juice	

FOOD FOR THE DAY	DESCRIPTION	
	Allowed	**Avoid**
OTHER	Homemade soups with fat-free broth or skim milk; gelatin desserts; angel food cake; pies, cake, or cookies made with allowed oils and egg substitute, egg whites, or allowed egg yolks; sherbet; simple puddings prepared with fruit juice or skim milk and egg substitute, egg whites, or allowed egg yolks; cocoa powder (not chocolate); nuts	Commercial soups; soups prepared with cream or whole milk; puddings, custards, and ice creams unless homemade with skim milk or nonfat dry milk; whipped cream desserts, whipped toppings; pies, cakes, and cookies unless homemade with allowed oils and egg yolks
	Sugar, syrup, honey; plain jelly and jam; gumdrops, hard candy	Candies made with chocolate, butter, or cream; commercially prepared popcorn
	All spices, seasonings, and flavorings	

Suggested Menu Plan for
Moderate Cholesterol/Fat Restricted Diet
(Select from foods described)

Breakfast
Fruit
Egg (no more than 4 yolks per week)
Cereal
Whole-grain bread
Margarine or oil (1–2 teaspoons)*
Skim milk
Hot beverage

Lunch or Supper
Lean meat or substitute (2–3 ounces)
Vegetable
Whole-grain bread
Margarine or oil (2 teaspoons)*
Fruit
Skim milk

Dinner
Lean meat or substitute (2–3 ounces)
Potato, pasta, or grain
Vegetable
Whole-grain bread
Margarine or oil (2 teaspoons)*
Fruit
Skim milk

---
*See List 6, Fat Exchanges, Section 4; may be used on bread, salads, or in cooking.

LOW SALT DIET
(No Added Salt)
(3000-4000 mg sodium [130-174 mEq])

Use: The Low Salt Diet (3000–4000 mg sodium) is useful in preventing or controlling edema and/or hypertension.

Adequacy: The suggested food plan provides foods in amounts that will provide quantities of nutrients (except iron for females) recommended by the NRC for the average adult.

Diet Principles:
1. Table salt (which is sodium chloride, containing about 40% sodium) and foods processed with salt are limited. Certain foods that contain liberal amounts of natural sodium and other foods that contain sodium compounds may be limited. The general diet is served without a salt packet and with the appropriate restrictions noted.
2. Some medications, including over-the-counter preparations for treatment of indigestion or excess acid, contain large amounts of sodium.
3. Salt substitutes may promote acceptance of sodium restricted diets, but should be used only if permitted by the physician or dietitian.

FOOD FOR THE DAY	FOOD TO LIMIT (FOODS HIGH IN SODIUM)
MILK	Buttermilk, instant cocoa mixes
MEAT and MEAT SUBSTITUTES	Smoked and salt cured meats or fish such as bacon, bologna, chipped beef, corned beef, frankfurters, ham, luncheon meats, pickled meats, salt pork, sausage, anchovies, caviar, pickled herring; regular canned tuna, salmon and sardines; cheese and most commercial entrees; (regular peanut butter in excess of 1 tablespoon per day)
FRUITS	None
VEGETABLES *(including potato)*	High sodium packaged potato products; sauerkraut; tomato juice or vegetable juices canned with salt

FOOD FOR THE DAY	FOOD TO LIMIT (FOODS HIGH IN SODIUM)
BREADS, CEREALS, and GRAINS	Breads, rolls, or crackers with salted toppings; pretzels with salt; high sodium frozen or packaged rice, macaroni, or noodle mixtures; salted popcorn; instant hot cereals
FATS	Salted gravy, bacon, salt pork, seasoned dips, salted nuts
FLUID	Commercially canned soups, bouillon, broths, or consommé, dehydrated soup mixes; bouillon cubes, granules, or packets
OTHER	Salt, seasoned salt, olives, pickles, relishes, meat tenderizer, flavor enhancer (MSG), meat sauces, steak sauce, soy sauce, Worcestershire sauce, catsup, chili sauce, imitation bacon bits, horseradish prepared with salt, prepared mustard, salt substitute, unless approved by physician or dietitian High sodium packaged mixes; packaged or frozen entrees; canned entrees; salted snack foods such as cheese puffs, corn chips, potato chips

Suggested Menu Plan for Low Salt Diet
(3000-4000 mg sodium [130-174 mEq])
(Select from foods described)

The suggested menu plan for the General Diet should be used with limitation of the foods listed above, which are high in sodium.

LOW SODIUM DIET
(2000 mg sodium [87 mEq])

Use: The Low Sodium Diet (2000 mg sodium) is useful in preventing or controlling edema and/or hypertension.

Adequacy: The suggested food plan provides foods in amounts that will provide quantities of nutrients (except iron for females) recommended by the NRC for the average adult.

Diet Principles:

1. All foods are prepared and served without salt, soda, or regular baking powder. Total servings of milk, meat, regular breads, cereals, and fats are controlled.
2. Some medications, including over-the-counter preparations for treatment of indigestion or excess acid, contain large amounts of sodium.
3. Local water supplies and water that has been chemically softened may contain considerable sodium. The amount of sodium in water should be determined and considered in menu planning.
4. Salt substitutes may promote acceptance of sodium restricted diets, but should be used only if permitted by physician or dietitian.

FOOD FOR THE DAY	DESCRIPTION	
	Allowed	**Avoid**
MILK *2-4 servings*	Up to 4 cups skim, low-fat, whole, or chocolate milk per day; 1 cup yogurt may be substituted for 1 cup milk if desired	Commercial cultured buttermilk, instant cocoa mixes, malted milk, milkshakes, milk mixes
MEAT and MEAT SUBSTITUTES *2 servings* *(total 4-6 ounces)*	Meat, fish, poultry, eggs, dried beans or peas, prepared or processed without salt; low sodium cheese or cottage cheese; low sodium peanut butter	Meat, fish, poultry, eggs processed or prepared with salt or sodium compounds; smoked salt cured meats or fish such as bacon, bologna, chipped beef, frankfurters, ham, luncheon meat, pickled meat, salt pork, sausage; anchovies, caviar, pickled herring, canned tuna, salmon, and sardines; shellfish such as clams, crabs, oysters, scallops, and shrimp; all cheese except low sodium cheese; regular peanut butter

FOOD FOR THE DAY	DESCRIPTION	
	Allowed	**Avoid**
FRUITS *2 or more servings*	All fruits and fruit juices	None
VEGETABLES *2 or more servings* *(including potato)*	Fresh, frozen, or unsalted canned vegetables except those listed to avoid Choices of fruits and vegetables should include a good source (or two fair sources) of vitamin C daily and a good source of vitamin A at least every other day.	Regular canned vegetables and vegetables juices, tomato sauce, sauerkraut and other vegetables in brine; canned hominy; potato chips; frozen, canned, or instant potatoes or substitutes to which salt or sodium compounds have been added
BREADS, CEREALS, and GRAINS *4 or more servings*	Regular yeast bread and rolls in limited amounts; quick breads made without salt, baking powder, or baking soda (low sodium baking powder may be used); crackers with unsalted tops; rusk; zwieback; Melba toast; tortilla shells; unsalted rice cakes; unsalted cooked whole-grain and enriched cereals; 1 serving per day of regular cooked or dry cereal; puffed wheat, puffed rice, shredded wheat, specially prepared low sodium cereals; whole-grain or enriched macaroni, spaghetti, noodles, or rice prepared without salt	Bread, rolls, or crackers with salted topping, quick breads Instant hot cereals, regular cooked or dry cereals in excess of 1 serving per day; canned, frozen, or prepackaged prepared rice, macaroni, or noodle mixtures
FATS *(in moderate amounts)*	Regular butter or margarine, salad oil, lard, or vegetable shortening; unsalted gravy; sour cream, low sodium mayonnaise, and salad dressing; low sodium peanut butter; unsalted nuts	Salted gravy, bacon, salt pork, seasoned dips, salted nuts

FOOD FOR THE DAY	DESCRIPTION	
	Allowed	**Avoid**
FLUID *6-8 cups*	Any homemade low sodium broth or soup made with allowed foods; low sodium commercial soups or bouillon; coffee, tea, or decaffeinated coffee; carbonated beverages, labeled as "very low sodium" (35 mg or less per serving)	All regular commercial broth, soup, bouillon, consommé (instant, canned, or frozen); carbonated beverages containing over 35 mg of sodium per serving
OTHER	Ice cream, sherbet, ice milk, pudding, or fruit-flavored yogurt when used as part of milk allowance; 1 serving per day of baked dessert made with salt, baking powder, or baking soda	Instant pudding mixes; baked desserts made with salt, baking powder, or baking soda in excess of 1 serving per day
	Spices and herbs, lemon juice, vinegar, cocoa powder, unsalted nuts, unsalted popcorn, and tortilla chips; low sodium catsup or mustard, low sodium pretzels or potato chips	Salt and salt-based seasonings such as celery salt, garlic salt, lemon pepper, meat tenderizer, monosodium glutamate, onion salt, seasoned salt, sea salt; barbecue sauce, meat sauce, catsup, chili sauce, prepared mustard, horseradish; pickles; olives; salted snack foods such as popcorn, nuts, corn chips, or pretzels
		Packaged mixes; packaged or frozen entrees; canned entrees

Suggested Menu Plan for Low Sodium Diet
(2000 mg sodium [87 mEq])
(Select from foods described)

Breakfast
Fruit or juice
Cereal with milk and/or egg
Whole-grain bread or toast with
  margarine or butter
Hot beverage

Lunch or Supper
Soup or juice, if desired
Meat or meat substitute
Vegetable
Whole-grain bread with
  margarine or butter
Fruit or allowed desserts
Milk

Dinner
Meat or meat substitute
Potato, pasta, or grain
Vegetable, cooked
Vegetable or fruit salad
Whole-grain bread with
  margarine or butter
Fruit or allowed dessert
Milk

PROTEIN RESTRICTED DIET
(40 g protein)

Use: The Protein Restricted Diet may be prescribed in certain stages of liver and kidney diseases where protein intakes need to be restricted.

Adequacy: This diet will not meet the dietary allowances for protein, iron, calcium, thiamin, riboflavin, niacin, and vitamin D recommended by the NRC.

Diet Principles:
1. Fifty to 70 percent of the total protein should be of high biological value (such as that found in eggs, milk, and meat). To be best utilized, this protein intake should be distributed throughout the day rather than at one meal.
2. The remaining protein can be provided by the lower quality protein found in breads, cereals, grains, and vegetables.
3. Adequate calorie intake is essential to ensure protein is used for tissue growth or repair rather than for energy needs. Additional calories may be incorporated through the use of sweetened fruit juice; high calorie, low protein formulas; low protein bread products; fats, and sugar.

Note: The diabetic exchange lists in Section 4 are used to calculate this diet.

FOOD FOR THE DAY	DESCRIPTION
MILK *1/2 cup*	Cream, milk (whole milk is recommended because of its greater calorie content)
MEAT *2 exchanges*	See Exchange List in Section 4. Meats may be coated with low protein flour or wheat starch and fried to increase calorie content. Milk and flour should not be used in meat preparation unless counted in the total day's protein allowance.
FRUITS *3 or more servings*	Fresh, frozen, canned, and dried fruits or juices can be used as desired. Sweetened products will increase caloric intake.

FOOD FOR THE DAY	DESCRIPTION
VEGETABLES *2 exchanges*	See Exchange List in Section 4. Fresh, frozen, or canned vegetables can be used. Fat may be used for seasoning, but milk and flour should not be added unless they are counted in the total day's protein allowance. Choices of fruits and vegetables should include a good source (or two fair sources) of vitamin C daily and a good source of vitamin A at least every other day.
BREADS, CEREALS, and GRAINS *6 exchanges*	See Exchange List in Section 4. For additional calories use additional low protein baked products. Low protein rusk and low protein bread are two examples. Wheat starch is also available for making other low protein baked goods.
FATS *5 teaspoons or more*	Fats are not limited and are an important source of calories. They can be used liberally in preparation and seasoning of foods.
FLUID *6-8 cups* *(unless restricted)*	Water and other fluids, such as coffee, tea regular carbonated beverages, fruit drinks (for example, Kool-aid), lemonade
OTHER	Sherbet, flavored gelatin, desserts made with wheat starch and other low protein products Custards, puddings, and pastries cannot be used unless the milk, egg, and flour are counted in the total day's protein allowance. Sweets are a good source of calories and can be used as desired: hard candies, jelly, jam, sugars, honey, syrups, popsicles, mints (no chocolate). Avoid the following sweets because of protein content: candy bars, caramels, chocolate candy, fudge, and peanut butter candy.

Suggested Menu Plan for Protein Restricted Diet
(40 g protein)
(Select from foods described)

Breakfast

	Fruit or juice
1/2 cup	Cereal
1 tablespoon	Sugar
1 slice	Whole-grain toast
1/2 teaspoon	Margarine or butter
1/2 cup	Whole milk
	Hot beverage

Lunch

1 ounce	Meat
1/2 cup	Vegetable
1/2 tablespoon	Margarine or butter
1 slice	Whole-grain bread
	Fruit
	Low protein dessert
	Hot beverage
1 tablespoon	Sugar, if desired
	Fruit juice

Midafternoon Snack

6 squares	Saltines
1/2 tablespoon	Margarine or butter
1–2 tablespoons	Jelly
	Fruit juice

Dinner

	Juice
1 ounce	Meat/Fish/Poultry
1/2 cup	Potato or substitute
1/2 cup	Vegetable
1 slice	Whole-grain bread
1/2 tablespoon	Margarine or butter
	Fruit
	Low protein dessert
	Hot beverage
1 tablespoon	Sugar, if desired

Evening Snack

	Fruit

LIBERAL RENAL DIET
(60-80 g protein, 3000 mg sodium, 3000 mg potassium, 1100 mg phosphorus)

Use: The Liberal Renal Diet is prescribed for persons with chronic renal insufficiency who require a moderate restriction of protein, sodium, potassium, and fluid. A more severe restriction should be calculated by a registered dietitian.

Adequacy: The suggested menu plan includes food in amounts that provide quantities of nutrients (except iron for females) recommended by the NRC for the average adult.

Diet Principles:
1. The suggested food plan provides 60–80 g protein and approximately 3000 mg sodium, 3000 mg potassium, and 1100 mg phosphorus, depending on number of servings and type of foods chosen.
2. Fluid limits should be individualized.
3. The Exchange Lists in Section 4 are used to define portion size and to calculate protein in this diet.
4. Guidelines for food selection on the Low Sodium Diet (2000 mg sodium) are followed to meet the sodium level.
5. Up to 1/4 teaspoon table salt (575 mg sodium) may be allowed daily to add at table.
6. Salt substitutes (potassium chloride) should not be used unless authorized by the physician. This will affect the potassium level of the total diet.
7. Potassium is calculated as 200 mg in each serving of fruits and vegetables but may actually be less. See Appendix table Potassium per Household Measure.
8. Care should be taken to provide needed calories.
9. The assistance of a dietitian is advisable in planning and individualizing this diet.

VALUES USED IN CALCULATING THE LIBERAL RENAL DIET

FOOD	AMOUNT	PROTEIN (g)	SODIUM (mg)	POTASSIUM (mg)	PHOSPHORUS (mg)
Milk	1 cup	8	120	340	240
Meat	1 oz	7	50	130	75
Starch/Bread	1 serving or 1/2 cup	3	150	50	45
Vegetables* (unsalted)	1/2 cup	2	10	200	40
Fruit	1 medium or 1/2 cup	–	–	200	15
Fats (salted)	1 tsp	–	50	–	–
Coffee or tea	1 cup	–	–	90	–

*Includes starchy vegetables

MEAL PATTERNS FOR LIBERAL RENAL DIETS

Protein Level	60 g	80 g
Total Food Servings		
Milk	1	1
Meat	4	6
Starch/Bread	6	8
Vegetables	3	3
Fruit	3	3
Fat	9	9
Coffee/Tea	2	2
Sodium (mg)	1700	2100
Potassium (mg)	2540	2900
Phosphorus (mg)	975	1215

Suggested Menu Plan for Liberal Renal Diet

The sample menu for the 1200 Calorie Diet in Section 4 can be adapted for the Liberal Renal Diet as follows:

1. Add two Starch/Bread servings per day for the 60 gram and four for 80 gram protein.
2. Use one less ounce meat for the 60 gram protein level and one more ounce for the 80 gram.
3. Add one vegetable serving. Treat potatoes, corn, and other starchy vegetables as a vegetable, not a starch/bread exchange.
4. Add six or more fat exchanges to increase calories.
5. Calories may also be increased through use of a carbohydrate supplement added to food or beverages. See Table of Products, Section 3.
6. Beverages and other liquids may be limited due to fluid restrictions.
7. Due to their high potassium content, do not serve dried beans, peas, lentils, or baked potato. Use only with a dietitian's guidance.

Suggested Menu Plan for Liberal Renal Diet

60 g Protein		*80 g Protein*
	Breakfast	
1/2 cup	Apple juice	1/2 cup
1/2 cup	Oatmeal	1/2 cup
1 slice	Toast with	2 slices
2 teaspoons	Margarine or butter	2 teaspoons
	Jelly	
1/2 cup	Milk, 2% or whole	1/2 cup
	Lunch or Supper	
2 slices	Bread for sandwich with	2 slices
1 ounce	Sliced roast beef	3 ounces
	Lettuce leaf	
1 teaspoon	Mayonnaise for sandwich	1 teaspoon
1/2 cup	Steamed carrots	1/2 cup
1 teaspoon	Margarine	1 teaspoon
1/2 medium	Apple	1/2 medium
	Dinner	
3 ounces	Baked fish	3 ounces
1/3 cup	Rice	2/3 cup
1/2 cup	Broccoli	1/2 cup
3 teaspoons	Margarine	3 teaspoons
1 cup	Tossed salad with	1 cup
2 teaspoons	Dressing	2 teaspoons
1/2 cup	Canned pineapple	1/2 cup
	Snack	
1/2 cup	Milk, 2% or whole	1/2 cup
3 squares	Graham crackers	3 squares
1/2 medium	Pear	1/2 medium

LACTOSE RESTRICTED DIET

Use: The Lactose Restricted Diet is used for persons who cannot digest lactose, the carbohydrate found in milk. Since the degree of sensitivity varies from person to person, the diet should be individualized.

Adequacy: The diet is adequate in all nutrients except calcium (and iron for females) as recommended by the NRC for the average adult. Calcium and vitamin D supplements may be advisable.

Diet Principles: The diet limits foods containing lactose according to individual tolerance. All labels should be read carefully to identify foods containing lactose, milk, milk solids, whey, or curd.

FOOD FOR THE DAY	DESCRIPTION	
	Allowed	**Include as Tolerated**
MILK *2 or more cups*	Soy milk and lactose-free milk substitutes; milk treated with lactase enzyme; e.g., Lactaid	Milk and milk products; (buttermilk and yogurt often tolerated)
MEAT and MEAT SUBSTITUTES *2 servings* *(total 4-6 ounces)*	All meat, poultry, fish, and shellfish; eggs; peanut butter, dried beans, lentils; cheeses with minimal lactose: blue, brick, Camembert, cheddar, Colby, Edam, provolone, Swiss, and pasteurized processed American	Any prepared with milk; cold cuts, wieners, or other meat with added lactose; other cheeses
FRUITS *2 or more servings*	All fruits and fruit juices	Fruit drinks containing lactose
VEGETABLES *2 or more servings* *(including potato)*	All vegetables and vegetable juices	Any prepared with milk or cheese sauce
BREADS, CEREALS, and GRAINS *4 or more servings*	Crackers, rusk, bread made without milk, Vienna or French bread; all cereals except those listed to avoid; rice, pasta, hominy, barley, cracked wheat	Any prepared with milk or milk products; instant cereals; dry cereals containing lactose or milk

FOOD FOR THE DAY	DESCRIPTION	
	Allowed	**Include As Tolerated**
FATS *in moderate amounts*	Milk-free margarine (Kosher or Pareve margarines do not contain milk); some nondairy cream substitutes (check label); vegetables oils, shortening, lard, bacon, salad dressings made without milk; peanut butter	Butter or margarine containing milk; salad dressings containing milk; mayonnaise-type salad dressings; sour cream, cream cheese, cream
FLUID *6-8 cups*	Broth-based soups, dried pea, bean and lentil soups; coffee, tea, soft drinks	Powdered soft drinks; drinks prepared with flavored instant coffees containing milk or lactose; cream soups, commercial soups containing milk or milk products
OTHER	Desserts made without milk; fruit ices, gelatin desserts; sugar, corn syrup, maple syrup, honey, jam, jelly, hard candies, marshmallows; most seasonings and flavorings	Any dessert, sauce, or mix containing milk or milk products; sherbet, ice cream, frozen yogurt; milk chocolate, caramels, cream or chocolate candies; artificial sweeteners containing lactose

Suggested Menu Plan for Lactose Restricted Diet

The menu plan for the General Diet should be used. Milk substitutes and milk-free foods as suggested above should be used where appropriate.

GLUTEN RESTRICTED DIET

Use: The Gluten Restricted Diet is used for persons with celiac disease or gluten-induced enteropathy.

Adequacy: The suggested food plan includes foods in amounts that will provide the quantities of nutrients (except iron for females) recommended by the NRC for the average adult. Optimal calories, protein, vitamins, and minerals should be provided since many patients may have malabsorption problems.

Diet Principles:
1. This diet avoids foods containing the protein, gluten, found in wheat, rye, oats, and barley grains.
2. Wheat starch, corn, rice, and products made from these grains may be used in place of the restricted grains.
3. It is important to carefully examine labels of all commercial and convenience foods to determine ingredients.
4. When long-term use of this diet is needed, a dietitian should assist in diet planning and teaching.

FOOD FOR THE DAY	FOODS TO AVOID (CONTAIN GLUTEN)
MILK *2 or more cups*	Commercial chocolate and malted milk drinks
MEAT and MEAT SUBSTITUTES *2 servings* *(total 4-6 ounces)*	Creamed or breaded meat, fish, or poultry unless made with allowed flours; commercial products containing the restricted grains; canned meat products; cold cuts unless all meat; cheese spreads
FRUITS *2 or more servings*	None
VEGETABLES *2 or more servings* *(including potato)*	Creamed or breaded vegetables
BREADS, CEREALS, and GRAINS *4 or more servings*	Any made with restricted grains; cooked and dry cereals made with restricted grains; pasta, macaroni, spaghetti, noodles, and others

FOOD FOR THE DAY	FOODS TO AVOID (CONTAIN GLUTEN)
FATS *in moderate amounts*	Salad dressings which contain gluten stabilizers; mayonnaise-type salad dressings
FLUID *6-8 cups*	Cereal beverages: Postum, Ovaltine, ale, beer; soups thickened or made with restricted grains
DESSERTS	Cakes, cookies, pastries, or pudding mixes; ice cream cones; ice cream or sherbet containing a wheat stabilizer

Suggested Menu Plan for Gluten Restricted Diet

Breakfast
Fruit or fruit juice
Egg
Rice or corn cereal
Low protein bread or rusk
Margarine
Milk
Coffee or tea

Lunch or Dinner
Meat or meat substitute
Potato, rice, or corn
Vegetable or salad
Rice cake
Margarine or salad dressing
Fruit, rice cookies, sherbet
Milk
Coffee or tea

Snacks
Any meat or cheese
Rice or corn crackers
Popped corn
Fruits
Vegetables
Milk

Summary Description of Diets

Name of Diet	Use	Adequacy
Bland	Treatment of chronic duodenal ulcer disease, hiatal hernia, and reflux esophagitis.	Provides the quantities of nutrients (except iron for females) recommended by the NRC for the average adult.
Calorie-controlled	Weight reduction or weight control.	With the exception of the 1000 Calorie Diet, provides the nutrients (except iron for females) recommended by the NRC for the average adult
Children	General diet for children aged 1-6 years.	Provides the quantities of nutrients (except for iron) recommended by the NRC for the average child.
Cholesterol/Fat Restricted (300 mg cholesterol; 30% calories from fat)	Reduction of cholesterol and fatty substances in the blood (hyperlipidemia).	Provides the quantities of nutrients (except iron for females) recommended by the NRC for the average adult.
Diabetic	Outline for planning a diet with a diabetic patient.	Provides the quantities of nutrients (except iron for females) recommended by the NRC for the average adult.
Dysphagia	For patients with neurogenic or myogenic swallowing or chewing difficulties.	Provides the quantities of nutrients (except iron for females) recommended by the NRC for the average adult.
Easily Chewed (mechanical soft)	Provides foods in a form that can be easily chewed and swallowed.	Provides the quantities of nutrients (except iron for females) recommended by the NRC for the average adult.

Fat, Low (40-50 g fat)	Treatment of diseases of gallbladder, liver, or pancreas, or if disturbances in fat digestion and absorption occur.	Provides the quantities of nutrients (except iron for females) recommended by the NRC for the average adult.
Fiber, High	Treatment of constipation, uncomplicated diverticulosis, irritable bowel syndrome or whenever a greater stool volume is desired; beneficial in blood glucose and blood lipid control.	Provides the quantities of nutrients (except iron for females) recommended by the NRC for the average adult.
Fiber, Low (low residue)	For patients receiving radiation therapy on or near the intestine, in partial bowel obstruction, in acute gastroenteritis, and in postoperative anal or hemorrhoidal surgery.	Provides the quantities of nutrients (except iron for females) recommended by the NRC for the average adult.
General	For persons who require no dietary modifications.	Provides the quantities of nutrients (except iron for females) recommended by the NRC for the average adult.
Geriatric, Liberal	For older persons as an alternative to more specific modified diets such as Diabetic, Low Salt, or Cholesterol/Fat restricted; for persons wanting a healthy alternative to the routine General Diet.	Provides the quantities of nutrients recommended by the NRC for the geriatric adult.
Gluten Free	Treatment of celiac disease or gluten-induced enteropathy.	Provides the quantities of nutrients (except iron for females) recommended by the NRC for the average adult. Optimal calories, protein, vitamins, and minerals should be provided since many patients have malabsorption problems.

High Calorie, High Protein, High Nutrient	For nutritional rehabilitation following a debilitating disease or surgery.	Provides calories, protein, minerals, and vitamins in amounts greater than recommended by the NRC for the average adult.
Infant	For infants from birth to 1 year who can take a regular diet.	Provides the quantities of nutrients recommended by the NRC for the average infant.
Lactose Restricted	For persons who cannot digest the milk sugar, lactose.	Provides the quantities of nutrients (except iron for females) recommended by the NRC for the average adult. Calcium and vitamin D supplements may be advisable.
Liquid, Clear	For preoperative or postoperative patients; in acute inflammation of the gastrointestinal tract; in acute stages of many illnesses; when it is necessary to minimize fecal material.	Inadequate in all nutrients. It should not be used more than two days without supplementation.
Liquid, Full	For the postoperative patient following clear liquids; for the acutely ill patient; for patients who cannot chew or shallow pureed or solid foods; to supplement a tube feeding.	Depending upon the amount and choice of food eaten, diet will tend to be low in protein, calories, iron, thiamin, and niacin. It is recommended for temporary use only. If used for more than two days, supplementation is necessary.
Postsurgical	For the postsurgical patient who is ready to have some solid foods but is not yet ready for a routine diet.	Depending upon the amount and choice of food eaten, this diet will tend to be low in protein, calories, iron, thiamin, and niacin. It is recommended for temporary use only.

Pregnancy and Lactation	Provides the increased amounts of protein, vitamins, and minerals needed by the pregnant or lactating woman.	Provides the quantities of nutrients (except iron and folacin) recommended by the NRC for the pregnant or lactating woman. Dietary supplements should provide only needed nutrients and should be taken only if prescribed by the physician.
Protein Restricted (40 g protein)	For persons who need to limit protein intake due to certain types of liver or kidney diseases.	Inadequate in protein, calcium, iron, thiamin, riboflavin, niacin, and vitamin D as recommended by the NRC for the average adult.
Pureed	For people who cannot chew or swallow more solid foods.	Provides the quantities of nutrients (except iron for females) recommended by the NRC for the average adult.
Renal, Liberal (60-80 g protein, 3000 mg sodium, 3000 mg potassium, 1100 mg phosphorus)	For patients with chronic renal insufficiency needing a moderate restriction of protein, sodium, potassium, phosphorus, and fluid.	Provides the quantities of nutrients (except iron for females) recommended by the NRC for the average adult.
Salt, Low (3000-4000 mg sodium [130-174 mEq])	For the prevention or control of edema and/or hypertension.	Provides the quantities of nutrients (except iron for females) recommended by the NRC for the average adult.
Sodium, Low (2000 mg sodium [87 mEq])	For the prevention or control of edema and/or hypertension.	Provides the quantities of nutrients (except iron for females) recommended by the NRC for the average adult.
Tube Feeding	For patients who are physically or psychologically unable to take food by mouth in amounts that will support adequate nutrition. Some of the described products may also be used as oral supplements.	Some tube feedings will be nutritionally adequate when given in recommended amounts, but it is important to evaluate each patient individually.

FOOD AND NUTRITION BOARD, NATIONAL ACADEMY OF SCIENCES—NATIONAL RESEARCH COUNCIL. RECOMMENDED DIETARY ALLOWANCES, Revised 1989

Designed for the maintenance of good nutrition of practically all healthy people in the United States

Category	Age (years) or Condition	Weight (kg)	Weight (lb)	Height (cm)	Height (in)	Protein (g)	Fat-Soluble Vitamins Vita-min A (µg RE)[c]	Vita-min D (µg)[d]	Vita-min E (mg α-TE)[e]	Vita-min K (µg)	Water-Soluble Vitamins Vita-min C (mg)	Thia-min (mg)	Ribo-flavin (mg)	Niacin (mg NE)[f]	Vita-min B6 (mg)	Fo-late (µg)	Vitamin B12 (µg)	Minerals Cal-cium (mg)	Phos-phorus (mg)	Mag-nesium (mg)	Iron (mg)	Zinc (mg)	Iodine (µg)	Sele-nium (µg)
Infants	0.0–0.5	6	13	60	24	13	375	7.5	3	5	30	0.3	0.4	5	0.3	25	0.3	400	300	40	6	5	40	10
	0.5–1.0	9	20	71	28	14	375	10	4	10	35	0.4	0.5	6	0.6	35	0.5	600	500	60	10	5	50	15
Children	1–3	13	29	90	35	16	400	10	6	15	40	0.7	0.8	9	1.0	50	0.7	800	800	80	10	10	70	20
	4–6	20	44	112	44	24	500	10	7	20	45	0.9	1.1	12	1.1	75	1.0	800	800	120	10	10	90	20
	7–10	28	62	132	52	28	700	10	7	30	45	1.0	1.2	13	1.4	100	1.4	800	800	170	10	10	120	30
Males	11–14	45	99	157	62	45	1,000	10	10	45	50	1.3	1.5	17	1.7	150	2.0	1,200	1,200	270	12	15	150	40
	15–18	66	145	176	69	59	1,000	10	10	65	60	1.5	1.8	20	2.0	200	2.0	1,200	1,200	400	12	15	150	50
	19–24	72	160	177	70	58	1,000	10	10	70	60	1.5	1.7	19	2.0	200	2.0	1,200	1,200	350	10	15	150	70
	25–50	79	174	176	70	63	1,000	5	10	80	60	1.5	1.7	19	2.0	200	2.0	800	800	350	10	15	150	70
	51+	77	170	173	68	63	1,000	5	10	80	60	1.2	1.4	15	2.0	200	2.0	800	800	350	10	15	150	70
Females	11–14	46	101	157	62	46	800	10	8	45	50	1.1	1.3	15	1.4	150	2.0	1,200	1,200	280	15	12	150	45
	15–18	55	120	163	64	44	800	10	8	55	60	1.1	1.3	15	1.5	180	2.0	1,200	1,200	300	15	12	150	50
	19–24	58	128	164	65	46	800	10	8	60	60	1.1	1.3	15	1.6	180	2.0	1,200	1,200	280	15	12	150	55
	25–50	63	138	163	64	50	800	5	8	65	60	1.1	1.3	15	1.6	180	2.0	800	800	280	15	12	150	55
	51+	65	143	160	63	50	800	5	8	65	60	1.0	1.2	13	1.6	180	2.0	800	800	280	10	12	150	55
Pregnant						60	800	10	10	65	70	1.5	1.6	17	2.2	400	2.2	1,200	1,200	320	30	15	175	65
Lactating	1st 6 months					65	1,300	10	12	65	95	1.6	1.8	20	2.1	280	2.6	1,200	1,200	355	15	19	200	75
	2nd 6 months					62	1,200	10	11	65	90	1.6	1.7	20	2.1	260	2.6	1,200	1,200	340	15	16	200	75

Source: *Recommended Dietary Allowances*, 10th revised edition, © 1989 by the National Academy of Sciences, National Academy Press, Washington, D.C.

[a] The allowances, expressed as average daily intakes over time, are intended to provide for individual variations among most normal persons as they live in the United States under usual environmental stresses. Diets should be based on a variety of common foods in order to provide other nutrients for which human requirements have been less well defined. See text for detailed discussion of allowances and of nutrients not tabulated.

[b] Weights and heights of Reference Adults are actual medians for the U.S. population of the designated age, as reported by NHANES II. The median weights and heights of those under 19 years of age were taken from Hamill et al. (1979) (see pages 16–17). The use of these figures does not imply that the height-to-weight ratios are ideal.

[c] Retinol equivalents. 1 retinol equivalent = 1 µg retinol or 6 µg β-carotene. See text for calculation of vitamin A activity of diets as retinol equivalents.

[d] As cholecalciferol. 10 µg cholecalciferol = 400 IU of vitamin D.

[e] α-Tocopherol equivalents. 1 mg d-α tocopherol = 1 α-TE. See text for variation in allowances and calculation of vitamin E activity of the diet as α-tocopherol equivalents.

[f] 1 NE (niacin equivalent) is equal to 1 mg of niacin or 60 mg of dietary tryptophan.

DESIRABLE WEIGHTS

Weight in pounds according to frame (in indoor clothing)

	Height Feet	Inches	Small Frame	Medium Frame	Large Frame
Men	5	2	128–134	131–141	138–150
of ages 25	5	3	130–136	133–143	140–153
and over	5	4	132–138	135–145	142–156
	5	5	134–140	137–148	144–160
	5	6	136–142	139–151	146–164
	5	7	138–145	142–154	149–168
	5	8	140–148	145–157	152–172
	5	9	142–151	148–160	155–176
	5	10	144–154	151–163	158–180
	5	11	146–157	154–166	161–184
	6	0	149–160	157–170	164–188
	6	1	152–164	160–174	168–192
	6	2	155–168	164–178	172–197
	6	3	158–172	167–182	176–202
	6	4	162–176	171–187	181–207

	Height Feet	Inches	Small Frame	Medium Frame	Large Frame
Women	4	10	102–111	109–121	118–131
of ages 25	4	11	103–113	111–123	120–134
and over	5	0	104–115	113–126	122–137
	5	1	106–118	115–129	125–140
	5	2	108–121	118–132	128–143
	5	3	111–124	121–135	131–147
	5	4	114–127	124–138	134–151
	5	5	117–130	127–141	137–155
	5	6	120–133	130–144	140–159
	5	7	123–136	133–147	143–163
	5	8	126–139	136–150	146–167
	5	9	129–142	139–153	149–170
	5	10	132–145	142–156	152–173
	5	11	135–148	145–159	155–176
	6	0	138–151	148–162	158–179

Source: Metropolitan Life Insurance Company, 1983.
Note: Weights at ages 25-59 based on lowest mortality. Weight in pounds according to frame (in indoor clothing weighing 5 lbs. for men and 3 lbs. for women; shoes with 1″ heels).

AVERAGE WEIGHT OF AMERICANS AGED 65-94

Men

Height in Inches	Ages 65–69	Ages 70–74	Ages 75–79	Ages 80–84	Ages 85–89	Ages 90–94
61	128–156	125–153	123–151			
62	130–158	127–155	125–153	122–148		
63	131–161	129–157	127–155	122–150	120–146	
64	134–164	131–161	129–157	124–152	122–148	
65	136–166	134–164	130–160	127–155	125–153	117–143
66	139–169	137–167	133–163	130–158	128–156	120–146
67	140–172	140–170	136–166	132–162	130–160	122–150
68	143–175	142–174	139–169	135–165	133–163	126–154
69	147–179	146–178	142–174	139–169	137–167	130–158
70	150–184	148–182	146–178	143–175	140–172	134–164
71	155–189	152–186	149–183	148–180	144–176	139–169
72	159–195	156–190	154–188	153–187	148–182	
73	164–200	160–196	158–192			

Women

58	120–146	112–138	111–135			
59	121–147	114–140	112–136	100–122	99–121	
60	122–148	116–142	113–139	106–130	102–124	
61	123–151	118–144	115–141	109–133	104–128	
62	125–153	121–147	118–144	112–136	108–132	107–131
63	127–155	123–151	121–147	115–141	112–136	107–131
64	130–158	126–154	123–151	119–145	115–141	108–132
65	132–162	130–158	126–154	122–150	120–146	112–136
66	136–166	132–162	128–157	126–154	124–152	116–142
67	140–170	136–166	131–161	130–158	128–156	
68	143–175	140–170				
69	148–180	144–176				

Source: Master, A. M., Lasser, R. P., and Beckman, G. 1960. Tables of average weight and height of Americans aged 65 to 94 years. *Journal American Medical Association* 172 (1960): 658. These tables also appear in *Des Moines Diet Manual,* 2d ed. 1981. Des Moines, Iowa: Central Iowa District Dietetic Association.

Note: Height is in stocking feet; weight includes light undergarments.

POTASSIUM PER HOUSEHOLD MEASURE

Food Groups	300 mg and More	100-300 mg
Dairy products	Fluid whole milk, lowfat milk, skim milk, butter-milk (8 oz) Nonfat dry milk solids (1/4 cup)	Ice cream (1 cup) Custard, baked (3/4 cup) Milk pudding, not canned (1/2 cup)
Meat, fish, poultry (3 oz cooked unless otherwise stated)	Beef Beef liver Chicken, light meat Pork, fresh, roasted Salmon, pink, canned Veal	Chicken, dark meat Frankfurter (1) Ham, cured Tuna, canned in oil White fish
Fruits and fruit juices (1/2 cup unless otherwise stated)	Apricots, dried*, cooked or uncooked Avocado* (1/2 medium) Banana (1 medium) Cantaloupe (1/2 medium) Dates, dried Figs, dried Honeydew melon (1/2 small) Peaches*, dried, cooked, or uncooked Prunes, dried, cooked, or uncooked Prune juice Raisins (1/4 cup) Watermelon* (1 slice, 6 in. [diameter × 1 1/2 in.])	Apple, raw (1 medium) Citrus juice, canned or frozen Fruit cocktail Grapefruit (1/2 medium) Orange, whole (1 medium) Papaya, fresh (1/3 medium) Peach, raw (1 medium) Pineapple juice (frozen or canned) Pomegranate, fresh (1 medium) Rhubarb, fresh, frozen, or cooked Strawberries, raw (1 cup) Tangelo (1 medium)
Vegetables, legumes, and vegetable juices (1/2 cup unless otherwise stated)	Beans, dry*, cooked Beet greens, cooked Mushrooms, fresh (10 small) Parsnips, raw or cooked Parsley* Peanut butter (3 tbsp) Potato, baked or boiled (1) Squash, winter, cooked Sweet potato, cooked (1 medium) Tomato, raw (1 medium) Tomato juice, canned (3/4 cup)	Broccoli, cooked Brussels sprouts, cooked Carrots, cooked Cauliflower, cooked Collards, fresh or frozen, cooked Kale, cooked Lentils, cooked Lettuce, raw (3 1/2 oz) Tomatoes, canned Vegetable juice cocktail (3/4 cup)

POTASSIUM PER HOUSEHOLD MEASURE

Food Groups	300 mg and More	100–300 mg
Breads and cereals (1/2 cup unless otherwise stated)	Bran cereal (100%) (1 cup)*	Apple pie (1/7 of 9 in. pie) Whole-grain cereals Bran Gingersnaps (10) Gingerbread (3 in. × 2 in. × 2 in.)
Other foods	Molasses, dark (2 tbsp) Yeast, brewer's (2 tbsp)	Cocoa (2 tbsp)

Source: Adapted from USDA Agricultural Research Service, Summer 1973.
*More than 500 mg potassium per common household measure. Revised, 1982.

SAFEGUARDS FOR FOOD

This diet manual will help in planning meals that will provide adequate nourishment for the sick and well alike. It is important that the food selected be safe. These safeguards will help prevent disease:

MILK	Use only pasteurized milk.
MEAT	Use only meat that has been inspected. The round stamp indicating federal inspection and the stamp indicating state inspection are guides to wholesome meat.
PORK and PORK PRODUCTS	Serve well cooked. An internal temperature of 170°F is adequate to produce safe pork. This is the only known way to prevent the disease trichinosis.
FRESH FRUITS and VEGETABLES	Wash thoroughly before cooking or serving raw. This helps to remove pesticides and other forms of contamination.
EGGS	Use only Grade A eggs. Buy no cracked or lower grade eggs. DO NOT SERVE UNCOOKED EGGS. These precautions are taken in an effort to prevent salmonellosis.
EGG PRODUCTS	Do not use egg products (liquid, frozen, or dried) unless they have been processed under the supervision of the U.S. Department of Agriculture and so labeled.
HOME CANNED FOODS	Do not serve in group care facilities. The risk of botulism is increased by use of these foods.
COOKED FOOD and LEFTOVERS	Refrigerate immediately in covered shallow containers. Discard small amounts of leftovers. Food that is not to be used within 24 hours should be frozen promptly.
FROZEN FOODS	Meat, fish, and poultry are to be thawed in the refrigerator, not at room temperature. Fruits and vegetables need not be thawed before cooking; allow extra time for preparation.

REFERENCES

Adams, Catherine F. 1975. *Nutritive values of American foods in common units.* USDA Agriculture Handbook 456. Washington, D.C.: U.S. Government Printing Office.

American Academy of Pediatrics. 1979. *Pediatric nutrition handbook.* Evanston, Ill.: AAP.

American Dietetic Association. 1981. *Handbook of clinical dietetics.* Chicago: ADA.

_____, 1986. *Exchange lists for meal planning.* Prepared by the American Dietetic Association and the American Diabetes Association. Chicago: ADA.

Anderson, L., et al. 1982. *Nutrition in health and disease.* 17th ed. Philadelphia: J. B. Lippincott.

Brody, Jane. 1982. *Jane Brody's nutrition book.* New York: Bantam Books.

Cataldo, C. B., et al. 1989. *Nutrition and diet therapy.* 2d ed. St. Paul: West Publishing Company.

Central Iowa District Dietetic Association. In Press. *The Des Moines diet manual.* 3d ed. Des Moines: CIDDA.

Krause, M. V., and L. K. Mahan. 1984. *Food, nutrition and diet therapy.* 7th ed. Philadelphia: W. B. Saunders.

Luros, E. 1981. A rational approach to geriatric nutrition. In *Ross Dietetic Currents,* vol. 8, no. 6. Columbus, Ohio: Ross Laboratories.

National Academy of Sciences, Food and Nutrition Board, Committee on Nutrition of Mother and Preschool Child. 1981. *Nutrition services in perinatal care.* Washington, D.C.: NAS.

National Dairy Council. 1985. *How to eat for good health.* Rosemont, Ill: NDC.

National Live Stock and Meat Board. 1987. *A food guide for the first five years.* Chicago: NLSMB.

National Research Council, Food and Nutrition Board, Subcommittee on the Tenth Edition of the RDAs. 1989. *Recommended Dietary Allowances,* 10th ed. Washington, D.C.: National Academy Press.

Pemberton, C. M., et al. 1988. *Mayo Clinic diet manual.* 6th ed. St. Louis: C. V. Mosby.

Pennington, Jean A. T. 1989. *Food values of portions commonly used.* 15th ed. New York: Harper and Row.

University of Iowa Hospitals and Clinics. 1989. *Recent advances in therapeutic diets.* 4th ed. Ames: Iowa State University Press.

U.S. Department of Agriculture. 1981. *Nutritive value of foods.* Home and Garden Bulletin 72. Washington, D.C.: U.S. Government Printing Office.

_____, 1985. *Nutrition and your health: Dietary quidelines for Americans.* Home and Garden Bulletin 232. Washington, D.C.: U.S. Government Printing Office.

USDA Agricultural Research Service. *Family economic review.* Summer 1973. Washington, D.C: U.S. Government Printing Office.

Williams, S. R. 1989. *Nutrition and dietary therapy.* 6th ed. St. Louis, Mo.: C. V. Mosby.